BIOCHEMISTRY and CLINICAL PATHOLOGY

PRACTICAL NOTEBOOK

for

FIRST YEAR DIPLOMA IN PHARMACY

(Also useful for students of B.Pharm and MBBS)

(According to new syllabus as prescribed by Pharmacy Council of India, Education Regulation 1991, implemented in the year 1993, for Diploma in Pharmacy Students)

Name: Mr / Ms. ______________________________

Class: D Pharma I yr ______________ Roll No: ______________

Subject: Biochemistry and Clinical Pathology Practical

Institution: ______________________________

BIOCHEMISTRY and CLINICAL PATHOLOGY

PRACTICAL NOTEBOOK

for

FIRST YEAR DIPLOMA IN PHARMACY

(Also useful for students of B. Pharm and MBBS)

(According to the new syllabus as prescribed by Pharmacy Council of India, Education Regulation 1991, implemented in the year 1993, for Diploma in Pharmacy Students)

Varun Dutt Sharma M. Pharm
Principal
and
Sudhir Kumar Pandey B. Pharm
Sr. Lecturer
Janta Polytechnic, Jahangirabad
Bulandshahar, Uttar Pradesh

CBS

CBS Publishers & Distributors Pvt. Ltd.

New Delhi • Bengaluru • Chennai • Kochi • Kolkata • Mumbai
Hyderabad • Nagpur • Patna • Pune • Vijayawada

ISBN: 978-81-239-1478-7

First Edition: 2007
Reprint: 2010, 2014, 2016, 2018, 2019, 2021

Published by **Satish Kumar Jain** and produced by **Varun Jain** for
CBS Publishers & Distributors Pvt. Ltd.,
4819/XI Prahlad Street, 24 Ansari Road, Daryaganj, New Delhi - 110002
delhi@cbspd.com, cbspubs@airtelmail.in • www.cbspd.com
Ph.: 23289259, 23266861, 23266867 • Fax: 011-23243014

Corporate Office: 204 FIE, Industrial Area, Patparganj, Delhi - 110 092
Ph: 49344934 • Fax: 011-49344935
E-mail: publishing@cbspd.com • publicity@cbspd.com

Branches:
- ***Bengaluru:*** 2975, 17th Cross, K.R. Road, Bansankari 2nd Stage, Bengaluru - 70 • Ph: +91-80-26771678/79 • Fax: +91-80-26771680 E-mail: cbsbng@gmail.com, bangalore@cbspd.com
- ***Chennai:*** No. 7, Subbaraya Street, Shenoy Nagar, Chennai - 600030 Ph: +91-44-26681266, 26680620 • Fax: +91-44-42032115 E-mail: chennai@cbspd.com
- ***Kochi:*** Ashana House, 39/1904, A.M. Thomas Road, Valanjambalam, Ernakulum, Kochi • Ph: +91-484-4059061-65 Fax: +91-484-4059065 • E-mail: cochin@cbspd.com
- ***Kolkata:*** 6-B, Ground Floor, Rameshwar Shaw Road, Kolkata - 700014 Ph: +91-33-22891126/7/8 • E-mail: kolkata@cbspd.com
- ***Mumbai:*** 83-C, Dr. E. Moses Road, Worli, Mumbai - 400018 Ph: +91-9833017933, 022-24902340/41 • E-mail: mumbai@cbspd.com

Representatives:
- Hyderabad: 0-9885175004
- Patna: 0-9334159340
- Jharkhand: 0-9811541605
- Nagpur: 0-9021734563
- Pune: 0-9623451994
- Uttarakhand: 0-9716462459

Printed at:
India Binding House, Noida, U.P.

Certificate

Student's Name ____________________

Class ____________________ Roll No. ____________

Subject ____________________

This is to certify that experiments, written in the index, have been performed by the student, are satisfactory.

Grade..................

Name and signature of teacher

College stamp

Date ....

Dedicated To Our Parents

Preface

The ultimate objective of technical education is to develop relevant skills, creativity and competence among the students so as to enable them to perform the task effectively and efficiently later in the world of work. Practical work consists of tasks that require some manipulation of apparatus or some action.

To achieve the above aim and to reduce the writing workload to some extent for the students, this PRACTICAL NOTEBOOK **of Biochemistry and Clinical Pathology** for first year diploma in pharmacy has been written according to the new syllabus prescribed by the Pharmacy Council of India, Education Regulation, 1991. This practical notebook contains 44 exercises, well illustrated with observation tables and normal clinical values to make more meaningful and serve as a guide to the students. A few blank pages are provided at end of this manual so that student can use these pages for writing additional experiments guided by the teachers depending on the availability of reagents and infrastructure of the concerned laboratory.

We express sincere thanks to Mr Satish Kumar Jain, Managing Director, and Mr YN Arjuna, Publishing Director, CBS Publishers & Distributors, New Delhi, for their cooperation, encouragement and assistance in bringing out this NOTEBOOK in its present form. Finally our greatest gratitude is to our colleagues and Mr Sandeep Kumar for his sincere cooperation in computer typing and setting the script.

We shall gratefully acknowledge the comments, suggestions and criticism by the teachers and students for improvement of future editions of this book.

Authors

Syllabus

PRACTICAL (75 hours)

1. Detection and identification of proteins, amino acids, carbohydrates and lipids.
2. Analysis of normal and abnormal constituents of blood and urine (glucose, urea, creatine, creatinine, cholesterol, alkaline phosphates, acid phosphates, bilirubin, SGPT, SGOT, calcium, diastase, lipase).
3. Examination of sputum and faeces (microscopic and staining).
4. Practice in injecting drugs by intramuscular, subcutaneous and intravenous routes. Withdrawal of blood samples.

List of Equipment for Biochemistry and Clinical Pathology Laboratory

	No. required for 60 students	No. required for 120 students
1	2	3
A. Special equipment and instruments		
1. Colorimeter	2	2
2. Microscopes	20	20
3. Permanent slides (skin, kidney, pancreas, smooth –muscle, liver, etc.)	Adequate	Adequate
4. Watch glasses	25	50
5. Centrifuge	1	1
6. Microscope with oil immersion.	5	5
B. General glassware	Adequate	Adequate
C. Biochemical reagents for analysis of normal and pathological constituents of urine and blood and facilities.	Adequate	Adequate

Contents

Instructions

1. In the laboratory student must be in uniform and should maintain strict discipline.
2. Always put on neat and clean white apron whenever you are working in laboratory.
3. Always bring practical notebook for viva and counter signature.
4. The practical notebook should be completed same day in every respect and should be submitted on the same day to the teacher concerned for the marking and signature.
5. Procedures are written in the language of students and procedûre written should be strictly followed.
6. Actual observations and readings should be recorded in the practical notebook; calculations and conclusions should be based on the actual observations.
7. Practical must be performed individually.
8. Safety rules must be followed strictly and student must know emergency treatment for accidents, laboratory infections, etc.
9. Keep your working place neat and clean.
10. Student must handle equipment, glassware and appliances carefully. Thoroughly clean the apparatus required in the practical work.
11. After the work is finished, the student should clean the apparatus and other articles.
12. Never take or use any chemical or reagents without the prior permission of teacher or lab. technician.
13. The physiological solution and working solution of drug should be prepared freshly at the time of conducting experiment.
14. The stock solution of the drugs can be stored under conditions specified individually.
15. Do not weigh less than 10 mg on a high quality analytical balance. For less than 10 mg of weighing of the any drug; it is advisable to prepare its solution by dilution method.
16. Never throw waste papers and burnt matchsticks in the sink; this will block the sink that may lead to overflowing. Put the waste materials in the dustbin.
17. The water taps and gas taps should be tightly closed after the work is over.
18. Electrical switches should be put off before leaving the laboratory.

INDEX

S. No.	Experiment	Date	Page No.	Remark

INDEX

S. No.	Experiment	Date	Page No.	Remark

INDEX

S. No.	Experiment	Date	Page No.	Remark

INDEX

S. No.	Experiment	Date	Page No.	Remark

1

Carbohydrates

Biochemistry

It is the branch of biology in which we study the biology at molecular level and equally it is the branch of organic chemistry in which we study the chemistry of living system.

Carbohydrates

These are compounds of carbon, hydrogen and oxygen. Previously, it was assumed that carbohydrates are hydrates of carbon but now defined, as carbohydrates are polyhdroxy aldehydes, polyhdroxy ketones or compound that can be hydrolyzed to them.

Classification

As per chemical structure

i. ***Monosaccharide***: Carbohydrates that cannot be hydrolyzed to simpler compounds. These are normally sweets and soluble in water.
   - ❖ The monosaccharide containing aldehyde group are called **aldose,** e.g. glucose.
   - ❖ The monosaccharide containing a keto group called **ketose,** e.g. fructose.

ii. ***Disaccharide***: Carbohydrates that can be hydrolyzed to two monosaccharide molecules. These are normally sweets, crystalline and soluble in water, e.g. sucrose, maltose and lactose, etc.

iii. ***Oligosaccharides***: Carbohydrates that can be hydrolyzed to three to seven monosaccharide, e.g. raffinose, rhamminose, etc.

iv. ***Polysaccharide***: Carbohydrates that can be hydrolyzed to many monosacharide molecules. These are normally tasteless and insoluble in water.
   - ❖ *Homopolysaccharide*: Polysaccharide that gives only one type of monosaccharide on hydrolysis, e.g. starch, glycogen, cellulose, etc.
   - ❖ *Hetropolysaccharide*: Polysaccharide that give two or three type of monomers on hydrolysis, e.g. heparin.

As per physical nature

i. ***Sugars***: These are the compounds, which are sweet, crystalline and soluble in water, e.g. glucose, sucrose, maltose and lactose, etc.
   - ❖ *Reducing sugars*: These are the compounds, which reduces Fehling's (or Benedict's) or Tollens' reagent, e.g. all monosaccharides.
   - ❖ *Non-reducing sugars*: These are the compounds, which do not reduce Fehling's (or Benedict's) or Tollens' reagent, e.g. sucrose.

ii. ***Non-sugars***: These are the compounds, which are non-crystalline, tasteless and insoluble in water, e.g. starch, cellulose, etc.

Stepwise Details for Identification of given Sample of Carbohydrate

Step 1

Molisch Test

Carbohydrates, dehydrated with conc. Sulphuric acid produce furfural or its derivative which on addition of ά-naphthol produce violet colour. If this test is positive means carbohydrates are present.

Step 2

Solubility Test: To the given sample add water.

- If soluble (Monosaccharide and disaccharides) e.g. glucose, fructose, lactose, maltose, sucrose, etc.
- If not soluble (Polysaccharide) e.g. starch, glycogen, etc.

Step 3 (A)

Reducing properties: Carbohydrates contain free carbonyl group act as reducing agent, such sugar are called reducing sugar and in polysaccharides and sugar like sucrose the carbonyl group attached to form glycoside bond, such carbohydrates are called non-reducing. To confirm this following tests are performed.

Fehling's test, Tommer's test, and Benedict's test: Reducing sugar reduces the cu++ ions present in the alkaline solution copper sulphate and produce coloured precipitate.

- If above tests are not positive (Non-reducing sugar present) e.g. sucrose.
- If above tests are positive (Reducing sugar present) e.g. glucose, fructose, lactose, maltose, etc.

Step 4

Barfoed's test: This is the test for identification of monosaccharide. In presence of weak acid, monosaccharides reduce copper ion to produce precipitate.

- If above tests is positive (Monosaccharide present) e.g. glucose, fructose, etc.
- If above tests is not positive (Disaccharide present) e.g. lactose, maltose, etc.

Step 5(A)

(a) Seliwanoffs test: It contain freshly prepared solution of resorcinol in HCl.

(b) Dehydration or furfural test: Ketose on dehydration with sulphuric acid give furfural or it derivatives.

- If above tests is positive, i.e. red precipitate, (Monosaccharide ketose present) e.g. fructose.
- If above tests is not positive (Monosaccharide aldose present) e.g. glucose.

Step 5(B)

Osazone test: Reducing sugars on heating with phenyl hydrazine, produce yellow crystalline compounds called osazone. Specific shape of crystals are produced by different reducing sugars as given in the table no., e.g. lactose, maltose, xylose, etc.

- Crystals of lactosazone (Lactose present).
- Crystals of maltosazone (Maltose present).
- Crystals of xylosazone (Xylose present).

Step 3 (B)

Iodine Test: Iodine reacts with polysaccharides to form coloured complex.

- If blue colour—starch
- If brown or reddish purple colour which disappears on heating and reappears on cooling—dextrin.
- If pink colour—glycogen.
- If deep blue colour—amylose.
- If purple colour—amylopectin.

Specific Tests for Some Common Carbohydrates

For glucose

1. Sample sol. + Sod. hydroxide	Brown resinous
2. Sample sol. + Methylene blue + 1 ml sod. hydroxide sol.—Boil	Depolarization of solution
3. Sample sol. + 1 ml picric sol. + 1 ml sod. hydroxide sol.—Boil	Red colour produced

For lactose

1. Sample sol. + Ammonical silver nitrate sol.—Warm	Silver mirror

For sucrose

Inversion tests: Sample sol. + 5 drops conc. HCl. Boil for 3 minutes – cool – neutralize with sod. hydroxide and perform following test:	Positive

1. Fehling's test
2. Benedict's test
3. Tommer's test
4. Barfoed's test

For galactose

Sample sol. 2.0 ml + 2.0 ml conc. HCl, mix, add a few drops of phloroglucinol, boil on water bath, red colour will appear.

Reagents

1. Fehling's reagents

(a) *Fehling's solution A*

Dissolve 34.6 gm of copper sulphate in 500 ml distilled water.

(b) *Fehling's Solution B*

Dissolve 17.3 gm of sodium potassium tartrate and 50 gm of NaOH in 500 ml of distilled water. Both the solutions are mix in equal volumes when needed for use otherwise it will deteriorate if they are mix together and kept for longer time.

2. Benedict's reagent

Dissolve 173 gm of sodium citrate and 100 gm of anhydrous sodium carbonate in 800 ml hot distilled water. Dissolve 17.3 gm of copper sulphate ($CuSO_4$ 5 H_2O) in 100 ml distilled water. Add copper sulphate solution slowly to carbonate citrate solution with constant stirring. Make up the volume to 1 litre with distilled water.

3. Molisch reagent

5% W/V of α naphthol in 95% alcohol.

4. Tommer's reagent

1% W/V of copper sulphate solution in distilled water. Make alkaline with equal volume dilute NaOH solution.

5. Barfoed's reagent

Dissolve 6.6 gm of crystalline copper acetate in 100 ml of distilled water. Add 0.9 ml of glacial acetic acid.

6. Seliwanoff's reagent

Dissolve 50 mg of resorcinol in 33 ml of 33% HCl.

7. Iodine solution

Dissolve 20 gm KI and 12.7 gm iodine in one litre distilled water.

Experiment 1

OBJECT

To identify the given sample of carbohydrate (glucose).

S. no.	*Test*	*Observation*	*Inference*
A.	**Physical test**		
1.	Colour		
2.	Smell		
3.	Solubility		
B.	**Chemical test**		
1.	***Molish's test***: Aq. or alcoholic solution of substance + 10% alcoholic sol. of naphthol, shake, add conc. Sulphuric acid through side of test tube.		
2.	***Fehling's test:*** 2 ml Aq. solution of substance + 2 ml Fehling's sol. A + 2 ml Fehling's sol. B, boil.		
3.	***Benedict's test***: 3 ml Aq. solution of substance + 5 ml Benedict's reagent, boiling for 2 minutes.		
4.	***Tommer's test***: 3 ml Aq. solution of substance + 2 ml Tommer's reagent, boiling for 2 minutes.		
5.	***Seliwanoff's test***: 1 ml Aq. solution of substance + 3 ml Seliwanoff's reagent, boiling for 2 minutes.		

S. no.	*Test*	*Observation*	*Inference*
6.	***Dehydration or furfural test***: 2 ml Aq. solution of substance + 2 ml α-naphthol sol. (1% in alcohol) + 5 ml conc. HCl, boiling for 2 minutes.		
7.	***Osazone test***: 0.2 gm sample + 0.4 gm phenyl hydrazine hydrochloride + 0.6 gm sodium acetate + 4 ml water. Heat on water bath for 20 minutes. Cool and allow for crystallization and observe crystals under microscope.		
8.	***Iodine test***: Suspension of polysaccharide + 2 drops of iodine solution.		
9.	***Confirmation test***:		

Conclusion

The given sample is ....

Remarks

1. If Molish's test positive means given sample contains carbohydrate.
2. If Fehling's test, Benedict's test and Tommer's Test are positive, means given sample contains reducing sugar.
3. If Seliwanoff's test is negative means aldose (i.e. glucose) present and ketose (i.e. fructose) absent.
4. If iodine test is negative means polysaccharide absent.
5. If confirmatory test for glucose is positive, means glucose is confirmed in the given sample.

Experiment 2

OBJECT

To identify the given sample of carbohydrate (sucrose).

S. no.	*Test*	*Observation*	*Inference*
A.	**Physical test**		
1.	Colour		
2.	Smell		
3.	Solubility		
B.	**Chemical test**		
1.	***Molish's test***: Aq. or alcoholic solution of substance + 10% alcoholic sol. of naphthol, shake, add conc. Sulphuric acid through side of test tube.		
2.	***Fehling's test***: 2 ml Aq. solution of substance + 2 ml Fehling's sol. A + 2 ml Fehling's sol. B, boil.		
3.	***Benedict's test***: 3 ml Aq. solution of substance + 5 ml Benedict's reagent, boiling for 2 minutes.		
4.	***Tommer's test***: 3 ml Aq. solution of substance + 2 ml Tommer's reagent, boiling for 2 minutes.		
5.	***Seliwanoff's test***: 1 ml Aq. solution of substance + 3 ml Seliwanoff's reagent, boiling for 2 minutes.		

S. no.	*Test*	*Observation*	*Inference*
6.	***Dehydration or furfural test***: 2 ml Aq. solution of substance + 2 ml α-naphthol sol. (1% in alcohol) + 5 ml conc. HCl, boiling for 2 minutes.		
7.	***Osazone test***: 0.2 gm sample + 0.4 gm phenyl hydrazine hydrochloride + 0.6 gm sodium acetate + 4 ml water. Heat on water bath for 20 minutes. Cool and allow for crystallization and observe crystals under microscope.		
8.	***Iodine test***: Suspension of polysaccharide + 2 drops of iodine solution.		
9.	***Confirmation test***:		

Conclusion

The given sample is ....

Remarks

1. If Molish's test positive, means given sample contain carbohydrate.
2. If Fehling's test, Benedict's test and Tommer's Test are negative, means given sample contains non-reducing sugar.
3. If Barfoed's test is negative means monosccharide absent (i.e. glucose and fructose absent).
4. If iodine test is negative means polysaccharide absent.
5. If confirmatory test for sucrose is positive, means sucrose is confirmed in the given sample.

Experiment 3

OBJECT

To identify the given sample of carbohydrate (fructose).

S. no.	*Test*	*Observation*	*Inference*
A.	**Physical test**		
1.	Colour		
2.	Smell		
3.	Solubility		
B.	**Chemical test**		
1.	***Molish's test***: Aq. or alcoholic solution of substance + 10% alcoholic sol. of naphthol, shake, add conc. Sulphuric acid through side of test tube.		
2.	***Fehling's test***: 2 ml Aq. solution of substance + 2 ml Fehling's sol. A + 2 ml Fehling's sol. B, boil.		
3.	***Benedict's test***: 3 ml Aq. solution of substance + 5 ml Benedict's reagent, boiling for 2 minutes.		
4.	***Tommer's test***: 3 ml Aq. solution of substance + 2 ml Tommer's reagent, boiling for 2 minutes.		
5.	***Seliwanoff's test***: 1 ml Aq. solution of substance + 3 ml Seliwanoff's reagent, boiling for 2 minutes.		

S. no.	*Test*	*Observation*	*Inference*
6.	***Dehydration or furfural test*:** 2 ml Aq. solution of substance + 2 ml α-naphthol sol. (1% in alcohol) + 5 ml conc. HCl, boiling for 2 minutes.		
7.	***Osazone test*:** 0.2 gm sample + 0.4 gm phenyl hydrazine hydrochloride + 0.6 gm sodium acetate + 4 ml water. Heat on water bath for 20 minutes. Cool and allow for crystallization and observe crystals under microscope.		
8.	***Iodine test*:** Suspension of polysaccharide + 2 drops of iodine solution.		
9.	***Confirmation test*:**		

Conclusion

The given sample is ....

Remarks

1. If Molish's test positive, means given sample contain carbohydrate.
2. If Fehling's test, Benedict's test and Tommer's test are positive, means given sample contains, reducing sugar.
3. If Seliwanoff's test is positive means aldose (i.e. glucose) absent and ketos (i.e. fructose) present.
4. If iodine test is negative means polysaccharide absent.
5. If confirmatory test for fructose is positive, means fructose is confirmed in the given sample.

Experiment 4

OBJECT

To identify the given sample of carbohydrate (starch).

S. no.	*Test*	*Observation*	*Inference*
A.	**Physical test**		
1.	Colour		
2.	Smell		
3.	Solubility		
B.	**Chemical test**		
1.	***Molish's test***: Aq. or alcoholic solution of substance + 10% alcoholic sol. of naphthol, shake, add conc. Sulphuric acid through side of test tube.		
2.	***Fehling's test***: 2 ml Aq. solution of substance + 2 ml Fehling's sol. A + 2 ml Fehling's sol. B, boil.		
3.	***Benedict's test***: 3 ml Aq. solution of substance + 5 ml Benedict's reagent, boiling for 2 minutes.		
4.	***Tommer's test***: 3 ml Aq. solution of substance + 2 ml Tommer's reagent, boiling for 2 minutes.		
5.	***Seliwanoff's test***: 1 ml Aq. solution of substance + 3 ml Seliwanoff's reagent, boiling for 2 minutes.		

S. no.	Test	Observation	Inference
6.	***Dehydration or furfural test*:** 2 ml Aq. solution of substance + 2 ml α-naphthol sol. (1% in alcohol) + 5 ml conc. HCl, boiling for 2 minutes.		
7.	***Osazone test*:** 0.2 gm sample + 0.4 gm phenyl hydrazine hydrochloride + 0.6 gm sodium acetate + 4 ml water. Heat on water bath for 20 minutes. Cool and allow for crystallization and observe crystals under microscope.		
8.	***Iodine test*:** Suspension of polysaccharide + 2 drops of iodine solution.		
9.	***Confirmation test*:**		

Conclusion

The given sample is ....

Remarks

1. If Molish's test positive, means given sample contain carbohydrate.
2. If sample is insoluble in water means polysaccharide is present.
3. If iodine test is positive, i.e. blue colour obtained means polysaccharide (starch) is present.
4. If confirmatory test for starch is positive, means starch is confirmed in the given sample.

Experiment 5

OBJECT

To identify the given sample of carbohydrate.

S. no.	*Test*	*Observation*	*Inference*
A.	**Physical test**		
1.	Colour		
2.	Smell		
3.	Solubility		
B.	**Chemical test**		
1.	***Molish's test***: Aq. or alcoholic solution of substance + 10% alcoholic sol. of naphthol, shake, add conc. Sulphuric acid through side of test tube.		
2.	***Fehling's test***: 2 ml Aq. solution of substance + 2 ml Fehling's sol. A + 2 ml Fehling's sol. B, boil.		
3.	***Benedict's test***: 3 ml Aq. solution of substance + 5 ml Benedict's reagent, boiling for 2 minutes.		
4.	***Tommer's test***: 3 ml Aq. solution of substance + 2 ml Tommer's reagent, boiling for 2 minutes.		
5.	***Seliwanoff's test***: 1 ml Aq. solution of substance + 3 ml Seliwanoff's reagent, boiling for 2 minutes.		

S. no.	Test	Observation	Inference
6.	***Dehydration or furfural test*:** 2 ml Aq. solution of substance + 2 ml α-naphthol sol. (1% in alcohol) + 5 ml conc. HCl, boiling for 2 minutes.		
7.	***Osazone test*:** 0.2 gm sample + 0.4 gm phenyl hydrazine hydrochloride + 0.6 gm sodium acetate + 4 ml water. Heat on water bath for 20 minutes. Cool and allow for crystallization and observe crystals under microscope.		
8.	***Iodine test*:** Suspension of polysaccharide + 2 drops of iodine solution.		
9.	***Confirmation test*:**		

Conclusion

The given sample is ....

Remarks

Experiment 6

OBJECT

To identify the given sample of carbohydrate.

S. no.	*Test*	*Observation*	*Inference*
A.	**Physical test**		
1.	Colour		
2.	Smell		
3.	Solubility		
B.	**Chemical test**		
1.	***Molish's test***: Aq. or alcoholic solution of substance + 10% alcoholic sol. of naphthol, shake, add conc. Sulphuric acid through side of test tube.		
2.	***Fehling's test***: 2 ml Aq. solution of substance + 2 ml Fehling's sol. A + 2 ml Fehling's sol. B, boil.		
3.	***Benedict's test***: 3 ml Aq. solution of substance + 5 ml Benedict's reagent, boiling for 2 minutes.		
4.	***Tommer's test***: 3 ml Aq. solution of substance + 2 ml Tommer's reagent, boiling for 2 minutes.		
5.	***Seliwanoff's test***: 1 ml Aq. solution of substance + 3 ml Seliwanoff's reagent, boiling for 2 minutes.		

S. no.	*Test*	*Observation*	*Inference*
6.	***Dehydration or furfural test*:** 2 ml Aq. solution of substance + 2 ml α-naphthol sol. (1% in alcohol) + 5 ml conc. HCl, boiling for 2 minutes.		
7.	***Osazone test*:** 0.2 gm sample + 0.4 gm phenyl hydrazine hydrochloride + 0.6 gm sodium acetate + 4 ml water. Heat on water bath for 20 minutes. Cool and allow for crystallization and observe crystals under microscope.		
8.	***Iodine test*:** Suspension of polysaccharide + 2 drops of iodine solution.		
9.	***Confirmation test*:**		

Conclusion

The given sample is ....

Remarks

Experiment 7

OBJECT

To identify the given sample of carbohydrate.

S. no.	*Test*	*Observation*	*Inference*
A.	**Physical test**		
1.	Colour		
2.	Smell		
3.	Solubility		
B.	**Chemical test**		
1.	***Molish's test***: Aq. or alcoholic solution of substance + 10% alcoholic sol. of naphthol, shake, add conc. Sulphuric acid through side of test tube.		
2.	***Fehling's test***: 2 ml Aq. solution of substance + 2 ml Fehling's sol. A + 2 ml Fehling's sol. B, boil.		
3.	***Benedict's test***: 3 ml Aq. solution of substance + 5 ml Benedict's reagent, boiling for 2 minutes.		
4.	***Tommer's test***: 3 ml Aq. solution of substance + 2 ml Tommer's reagent, boiling for 2 minutes.		
5.	***Seliwanoff's test***: 1 ml Aq. solution of substance + 3 ml Seliwanoff's reagent, boiling for 2 minutes.		

S. no.	*Test*	*Observation*	*Inference*
6.	***Dehydration or furfural test*:** 2 ml Aq. solution of substance + 2 ml α-naphthol sol. (1% in alcohol) + 5 ml conc. HCl, boiling for 2 minutes.		
7.	***Osazone test*:** 0.2 gm sample + 0.4 gm phenyl hydrazine hydrochloride + 0.6 gm sodium acetate + 4 ml water. Heat on water bath for 20 minutes. Cool and allow for crystallization and observe crystals under microscope.		
8.	***Iodine test*:** Suspension of polysaccharide + 2 drops of iodine solution.		
9.	***Confirmation test*:**		

Conclusion

The given sample is ....

Remarks

2

Lipids

These are water insoluble organic substances, physically oily and greasy that can be extracted from cells by organic solvents such as ether and chloroform. Lipids provide insulation to the body against variation in temperature of weather. Lipids are also reserve source of energy during starvation. Structurally, lipids cover a diversify group of compounds like steroids, fatty acids and some vitamins.

Classification

Simple lipids

These are esters of fatty acids with alcohol.

i. ***Neutral***: Ester of fatty acids with glycerol.
   - Contain saturated fatty acids, e.g. stearic acid and palmitic acids, etc.
   - Contain unsaturated or essential fatty acids, e.g. linoleic acid and oleic acids, etc.
   - Triglycerides-containing three fatty acid molecules esterified with three-hydroxyl group of glycerol, e.g. tristerin.

ii. ***Waxes***: True wax., e.g. Bee's wax.

iii. ***Vitamins***: Vitamin A, vitamin D.

Compound lipids

These are esters of fatty acids with alcohol which contain other element functional group, e.g. phospholipids, glycerides, etc. (Glycerides when reacts with methanol in the presence of acid or basic catalyst, produce ***glycerols.***

Other

Like carotenoids, steroids (e.g. ***cholesterol***), vitamin D, ketone bodies, etc.

Stepwise Details for Identification of Simple Lipids

Physical tests

Step 1

Solubility test: Lipids are insoluble in water but soluble in organic solvents like chloroform, ether, etc. Take in separate test tubes 5 ml of water, 5 ml of ether and 5 ml of chloroform. Add 2 to 3 drops of sample of lipid to each test tube and observe. In chloroform and ether sample it miscible while it is immiscible with water and floats on water.

Step 2

Grease spot test: These are oily and greasy to touch sensation. Due to greasy nature lipids make a spot on filter paper. Dissolve sample in organic solvents like ether or chloroform and place a drop of the solution on a filter paper and wait for drying. A translucent stain appears on filter paper.

Step 3

Litmus test: Due to neutral nature so no change in colour of red litmus paper.

Step 4

Specific gravity test: Because specific gravity of fat is less than one so on addition of water to lipids, fats or fatty acids float on water.

Chemical tests

Step 1

Emulsification test: In this process dispersed phase (lipid/fatty material) is divided in to very small droplets and distributed uniformly in water (dispersion medium) to form an emulsion. A suitable emulsifying agent can be added to form a stable emulsion. To alcoholic solution of sample, add double quantity of water, shake vigorously. A white emulsion is formed which on standing separates in the form of oil droplets of dispersed phase (lipid/fatty material). A stabilizing or emulsifying agent like bile salt is added, a emulsion is produced which remain stable on standing.

Step 2

Saponification test: In this process fats are hydrolyzed by alcoholic solution of alkali hydroxide (potassium hydroxide, sod. hydroxide or calcium hydroxide) to produce soap. Fatty acids can produce soap directly with alkali). To 1 ml of alcoholic sample add 2 ml of 10% sodium hydroxide and boil very carefully on water bath till mixture do not separate when one drop of oil is added. A soft mass is produced which soon redissolves. To this add 15 ml water, divide the solution in three parts and perform following tests:

(a) To 3 ml of sol., add NaCl to saturate it. A white ppt. of soap is produced. Then add 5 ml of water, ppt. dissolves because sodium soap is soluble in water.

(b) To 3 ml of sol., add equal quantity of conc. HCl or H_2SO_4. Small drops of oil will be separated which floats on top of water because soap salt of fatty acid is converted in to insoluble fatty acid by addition of HCl or H_2SO_4.

(c) To 3 ml of sol., after neutralizing it add 2% $CaCl_2$ solution. A white ppt. of soap is produced because calcium soap is insoluble in water.

Step 3

Iodine absorption test: Unsaturated fatty acids react with iodine due to presence of double bond. To 5 ml solution of sample in chloroform, add Hubl's iodine (Iodine + Mercuric chloride) drop-wise with continuous shaking and observe. If solution decolorizes means unsaturated fatty acids are present.

Specific test for glycerol

Step 1

Formation acrolein test: Glycerol can be dehydrated from fat with the help of solid potassium bi-sulphate and acrylic aldehyde or acrolein is obtained which possess irritating odour. To 2 drops of glycerol add little $NaHSO_4$ in dry test tube, on heating irritating odour is produced.

Stepwise Details for Identification of other Lipids

Specific Test for Cholesterol

Step 1

Physical form of cholesterol: Cholesterol is a non-saponifiable lipid because it does not contain any fatty acid, so cannot produce soap. It contain basic steroidal nucleus, fat soluble and is found only in animals. It appears in the form of white crystals.

Step 2

Solubility test: Lipids are insoluble in water but soluble in organic solvents like chloroform, ether, etc. Take in separate test tubes 5 ml of water, 5 ml of ether and 5 ml of chloroform. Add 2 to 3 drops of sample of cholesterol to each test tube and observe. In chloroform and ether, cholesterol is miscible while it is immiscible with water and floats on water.

Step 3

Salkowski's test: To 2 ml sol. of cholesterol in chloroform add 2 ml conc. Sulphuric acid vary slowly and mix carefully. The upper layer of chloroform becomes red and lower layer of sulphuric acid changes to yellow with green flouresence.

Step 4

Liberman-Burchard's test: To 2 ml sol. of cholesterol in chloroform, add 10 drops of acetic anhydride and 2 drops of conc. Sulphuric acid very slowly and mix carefully. The rose red colour is obtained which rapidly changes to blue and finally to bluish green.

Experiment 8

OBJECT

To identify the given sample of simple lipid (fatty acid).

S. no.	*Test*	*Observation*	*Inference*
A.	**Physical test**		
1.	Colour		
2.	Smell		
3.	***Solubility test*:** Take separately 5 ml water, 5 ml ether and 5 ml chloroform in test tubes and to each test tube add 3-3 drops of sample.		
4.	***Grease spot test*:** A drop of solution of sample in chloroform or ether is placed on filter paper and is dried.		
5.	***Litmus test*:** A drop of solution of sample in chloroform or ether is placed on litmus paper and is dried.		
6.	***Specific gravity test*:** To 4 ml of sample, add 5 ml of water in a test tube and allow to stand.		
B.	**Chemical test**		
1.	***Emulsification test*:** To alcoholic solution of sample add double quantity of water, shake vigorously and allow to stand.		

S. no.	*Test*	*Observation*	*Inference*
2.	***Saponification test***: To 1 ml alcoholic sol. of sample, add 2 ml 10% sod. hydroxide, boil, add 15 ml water and perform following tests: (a) 3 ml sol., add NaCl to saturate (b) 3 ml sol., add 3 ml conc. HCl (c) 3 ml neutralized sol., add calcium chloride sol.		
3.	***Iodine absorption test***: To 5 ml solution of sample in chloroform, add Hubl's iodine drop-wise with continuous shaking.		
4	***Confirmation test***:		

Conclusion

The given sample is ....

Remarks

Experiment 9

OBJECT

To identify the given sample of simple lipid (fatty acid).

S. no.	*Test*	*Observation*	*Inference*
A.	**Physical test**		
1.	Colour		
2.	Smell		
3.	***Solubility test*:** Take separately 5 ml water, 5 ml ether and 5 ml chloroform in test tubes and to each test tube add 3-3 drops of sample.		
4.	***Grease spot test*:** A drop of solution of sample in chloroform or ether is placed on filter paper and is dried.		
5.	***Litmus test*:** A drop of solution of sample in chloroform or ether is placed on litmus paper and is dried.		
6.	***Specific gravity test*:** To 4 ml of sample add 5 ml of water in a test tube and allow to stand.		
B.	**Chemical test**		
1.	***Emulsification test*:** To alcoholic solution of sample add double quantity of water, shake vigorously and allow to stand.		

S. no.	*Test*	*Observation*	*Inference*
2.	***Saponification test***: To 1 ml alcoholic sol. of sample, add 2 ml 10% sod. hydroxide, boil, add 15 ml water and perform following tests: (a) 3 ml sol., add NaCl to saturate (b) 3 ml sol., add 3 ml conc. HCl (c) 3 ml neutralized sol., add calcium chloride sol.		
3.	***Iodine absorption test***: To 5 ml solution of sample in chloroform, add Hubl's iodine drop-wise with continuous shaking.		
4.	***Confirmation test***:		

Conclusion

The given sample is ....

Remarks

Experiment 10

OBJECT

To identify the given sample of simple lipid (fatty acid).

S. no.	*Test*	*Observation*	*Inference*
A.	**Physical test**		
1.	Colour		
2.	Smell		
3.	***Solubility test*:** Take separately 5 ml water, 5 ml ether and 5 ml chloroform in test tubes and to each test tube add 3-3 drops of sample.		
4.	***Grease spot test*:** A drop of solution of sample in chloroform or ether is placed on filter paper and is dried.		
5.	***Litmus test*:** A drop of solution of sample in chloroform or ether is placed on litmus paper and is dried.		
6.	***Specific gravity test*:** To 4 ml of sample add 5 ml of water in a test tube and allow to stand.		
B.	**Chemical test**		
1.	***Emulsification test*:** To alcoholic solution of sample add double quantity of water, shake vigorously and allow to stand.		

S. no.	*Test*	*Observation*	*Inference*
2.	***Saponification test*:** To 1 ml alcoholic sol. of sample, add 2 ml 10% sod. hydroxide, boil, add 15 ml water and perform following tests: (a) 3 ml sol., add NaCl to saturate (b) 3 ml sol., add 3 ml conc. HCl (c) 3 ml neutralized sol., add calcium chloride sol.		
3.	***Iodine absorption test*:** To 5 ml solution of sample in chloroform, add Hubl's iodine drop-wise with continuous shaking.		
4.	***Confirmation test*:**		

Conclusion

The given sample is ....

Remarks

Experiment 11

OBJECT

To identify the given sample of other lipid (cholesterol).

S. no.	*Test*	*Observation*	*Inference*
A.	**Physical test**		
1.	Colour		
2.	Smell		
3.	***Solubility test***: Take separately 5 ml water, 5 ml ether and 5 ml chloroform in test tubes and to each test tube add 3-3 drops of sample.		
4.	***Grease spot test***: A drop of solution of sample in chloroform or ether is placed on filter paper and is dried.		
5.	***Litmus test***: A drop of solution of sample in chloroform or ether is placed on litmus paper and is dried.		
6.	***Specific gravity test***: To 4 ml of sample add 5 ml of water in a test tube and allow to stand.		
B.	**Chemical test**		
1.	***Emulsification test***: To alcoholic solution of sample add double quantity of water, shake vigorously and allow to stand.		

S. no.	*Test*	*Observation*	*Inference*
2.	***Saponification test***: To 1 ml alcoholic sol. of sample, add 2 ml 10% sod. hydroxide, boil, add 15 ml water and perform following tests: (a) 3 ml sol., add NaCl to saturate (b) 3 ml sol., add 3 ml conc. HCl (c) 3 ml neutralized sol., add calcium chloride sol.		
3.	***Iodine absorption test***: To 5 ml solution of sample in chloroform, add Hubl's iodine drop-wise with continuous shaking.		
4.	***Salkowski's test***: To 2 ml sol. of cholesterol in chloroform add 2 ml conc. Sulphuric acid vary slowly and mix carefully.		
5.	***Liberman-Burchard's test***: To 2 ml sol. of cholesterol in chloroform add 10 drops of acetic anhydride and 2 drops of conc. Sulphuric acid vary slowly and mix carefully.		

Conclusion

The given sample is ....

Remarks

Experiment 12

OBJECT

To identify the given sample of other lipid.

S. no.	*Test*	*Observation*	*Inference*
A.	**Physical test**		
1.	Colour		
2.	Smell		
3.	***Solubility test*:** Take separately 5 ml water, 5 ml ether and 5 ml chloroform in test tubes and to each test tube add 3-3 drops of sample.		
4	***Grease spot test*:** A drop of solution of sample in chloroform or ether is placed on filter paper and is dried.		
5.	***Litmus test*:** A drop of solution of sample in chloroform or ether is placed on litmus paper and is dried.		
6.	***Specific gravity test*:** To 4 ml of sample add 5 ml of water in a test tube and allow to stand.		
B.	**Chemical test**		
1.	***Emulsification test*:** To alcoholic solution of sample add double quantity of water, shake vigorously and allow to stand.		

S. no.	*Test*	*Observation*	*Inference*
2.	***Saponification test***: To 1 ml alcoholic sol. of sample, add 2 ml 10% sod. hydroxide, boil, add 15 ml water and perform following tests: (a) 3 ml sol., add NaCl to saturate (b) 3 ml sol., add 3 ml conc. HCl (c) 3 ml neutralized sol., add calcium chloride sol.		
3.	***Iodine absorption test***: To 5 ml solution of sample in chloroform, add Hubl's iodine drop-wise with continuous shaking.		
4.	***Salkowski's test***: To 2 ml sol. of cholesterol in chloroform add 2 ml conc. Sulphuric acid vary slowly and mix carefully.		
5.	***Liberman-Burchard's test***: To 2 ml sol. of cholesterol in chloroform add 10 drops of acetic anhydride and 2 drops of conc. Sulphuric acid vary slowly and mix carefully.		

Conclusion

The given sample is ....

Remarks

Experiment 13

OBJECT

To identify the given sample of other lipid (glycerol).

S. no.	*Test*	*Observation*	*Inference*
A.	**Physical test**		
1.	Colour		
2.	Smell		
3.	***Solubility test*:** Take separately 5 ml water, 5 ml ether and 5 ml chloroform in test tubes and to each test tube add 3-3 drops of sample.		
4.	***Grease spot test*:** A drop of solution of sample in chloroform or ether is placed on filter paper and is dried.		
5.	***Litmus test*:** A drop of solution of sample in chloroform or ether is placed on litmus paper and is dried.		
6.	***Specific gravity test*:** To 4 ml of sample add 5 ml of water in a test tube and allow to stand.		
B.	**Chemical test**		
1.	***Emulsification test*:** To alcoholic solution of sample add double quantity of water, shake vigorously and allow to stand.		

S. no.	*Test*	*Observation*	*Inference*
2.	***Saponification test*:** To 1 ml alcoholic sol. of sample, added 2 ml 10% sod. hydroxide, boil, add 15 ml water and perform following tests: (a) 3 ml sol., add NaCl to saturate (b) 3 ml sol., add 3 ml conc. HCl (c) 3 ml neutralized sol., add calcium chloride sol.		
3.	***Iodine absorption test*:** To 5 ml solution of sample in chloroform, add Hubl's iodine drop-wise with continuous shaking.		
4.	***Copper sulphate test*:** To 1 ml of 5% copper sulphate sol., add 5 ml of sample and 5 drops of 5% NaOH sol.		
5.	***Borax test*:** To 5 ml of borax sol., add 4-5 drops of phenolphthalein and sample sol. was heated.		
6.	***Acrolein test*:** To 2 drops of glycerol add little $NaHSO_4$ in dry test tube, heat.		

Conclusion

The given sample is ....

Remarks

Experiment 14

OBJECT

To identify the given sample of other lipid.

S. no.	Test	Observation	Inference
A.	**Physical test**		
1.	Colour		
2.	Smell		
3.	***Solubility test*:** Take separately 5 ml water, 5 ml ether and 5 ml chloroform in test tubes and to each test tube add 3-3 drops of sample.		
4.	***Grease spot test*:** A drop of solution of sample in chloroform or ether is placed on filter paper and is dried.		
5.	***Litmus test*:** A drop of solution of sample in chloroform or ether is placed on litmus paper and is dried.		
6.	***Specific gravity test*:** To 4 ml of sample add 5 ml of water in a test tube and allow to stand.		
B.	**Chemical test**		
1.	***Emulsification test*:** To alcoholic solution of sample add double quantity of water, shake vigorously and allow to stand.		

S. no.	*Test*	*Observation*	*Inference*
2.	***Saponification test***: To 1 ml alcoholic sol. of sample, add 2 ml 10% sod. hydroxide, boil, added 15 ml water and perform following tests: (a) 3 ml sol., add NaCl to saturate (b) 3 ml sol., add 3 ml conc. HCl (c) 3 ml neutralized sol., add calcium chloride sol.		
3.	***Iodine absorption test***: To 5 ml solution of sample in chloroform, add Hubl's iodine drop-wise with continuous shaking.		
4.	***Copper sulphate test***: To 1 ml of 5% copper sulphate sol., add 5 ml of sample and 5 drops of 5% NaOH sol.		
5.	***Borax test***: To 5 ml of borax sol., add 4-5 drops of phenolphthalein and sample sol. was heated.		
6.	***Acrolein test***: To 2 drops of glycerol add little $NaHSO_4$ in dry test tube, heat.		

Conclusion

The given sample is ....

Remarks

3

Amino Acids and Proteins

AMINO ACIDS

These are basically α-amino carboxylic acids, represented by general formula $H_2N\text{-}CHR\text{-}COOH$, the amino group attached to α position of carbon. These are the monomers or basic unit of proteins. These are non-volatile crystalline solids, soluble in water but insoluble in organic solvents like ether, benzene, etc. Total 26 amino acids are found in proteins in which 20 amino acids are prepared in living cell and called standard or basic amino acids, e.g. cystine, glutamine, etc. and other must be fed to the body for proper growth because these are not synthesized in the body, called essential amino acids, e.g. arginine, leucine, etc.

Classification

- *Non-polar, aliphatic*: e.g. glycine, alanine.
- *Polar, aliphatic*: e.g. glutamine, threonine, etc.
- *Aromatic*: e.g. tyrocine.
- *Contain sulpher*: e.g. cysteine.
- *Contain secondary amino group*: e.g. proline.
- *Acidic amino acids*: e.g. glutamate.
- *Basic amino acids*: e.g. lysine.

PROTEINS

Chemically, these are high polymers (polymers of α-amino acids where α-amino acids are polymerized by formation of number of peptide linkages), polyamides, nitrogenous, highly complex substances, occur in all living systems usually contain carbon, hydrogen, oxygen and sulpher, other elements like phosphorus and iron may also be present. These are optically active and amphoteric in character. These are complex macromolecular substances made up of amino acids. A single molecule of protein may contain hundreds or even thousands units of amino acids thus forming infinite combinations.

Classification

Broadly can be divided as follows

i. ***Fibrous proteins***: These are insoluble in common solvents, but are soluble in strong acids and alkalis. These are chief structural materials of animal tissues, e.g. keratin protein in skin, hair and nails, etc. collagen protein in tendons and myosin protein in muscles.
ii. ***Corpuscular or globular proteins***: These are soluble in water and aqueous solutions acids, alkalis and salts and forming colloidal solution due to large size of protein molecule. These are essential to maintain and

regulate the life process. They make all enzymes, many hormones like insulin, antibodies and hemoglobin in blood, albumin in eggs.

According to nutrition value can be divided as follows

i. ***Complete nutrition proteins***: These contains all essential amino acids, e.g. caseinogens protein in milk and albumin proteins in egg.
ii. ***Incomplete nutrition proteins***: Not containing all essential amino acids, e.g. gelatin, zein of maize.

According to function can be divided as follows

i. ***Enzymes***: Catalyze all biochemical reactions.
ii. ***Transport proteins***: Function is to carry metabolites gasses, e.g. hemoglobin.
iii. ***Regulatory proteins***: Controls metabolic activity, e.g. some hormones like insulin.
iv. ***Defense proteins***: Protect life against infection, e.g. antibodies.
v. ***Structural proteins***: Required to provide strength to cells and tissues, e.g. collagen protein of skin.

Systematically can be divided as follows

i. ***Simple proteins***: These are made up of peptide chains and on hydrolysis produce only amino acids.
   - *Albumins*: Soluble in water, acids and alkalis, coagulated by heat, e.g. serum albumin, egg albumin.
   - *Globulins*: Insoluble in water but soluble in acids and alkalis, coagulated by heat, e.g. serum globulin and vegetable globulin.
   - *Prolamines*: Insoluble in water but soluble in acids and alkalis, also soluble in alcohol, e.g. zein (from maize), gliadin (from wheat).
   - *Gelutenis*: Insoluble in water but soluble in acids and alkalis, coagulated by heat, e.g. gelutenin (from wheat), oryzenin (from rice).
   - *Albuminoids or sclero proteins*: Insoluble in water but soluble in strong acids and alkalis, e.g. keratin (from hair), fibroin (from silk), collagens (in skin, bones) which form gelatin (a water soluble protein) on boiling, Elastins (in tendons and arteries).
   - *Basic proteins*: These are strongly basic in nature and can be further divided as follows:
     a. **Histones:** Soluble in water, dilute acids and alkalies but insoluble in dilute ammonia, not coagulated by heat. These are proteins of nucleic acids, hemoglobin, etc.
     b. **Protamines:** These are stronger basic than histones. Soluble in water, dilute ammonia acids and alkalis, e.g. salmine of sperm.

ii. ***Conjugated proteins***: These contain a non-peptide portion (called prosthetic group which is responsible for specific biological activity of protein) attached to the protein part. These can be sub-divided as:
   - *Nucleoproteins*: Prosthetic group is nucleic acid.
   - *Chromoproteins*: Metal like iron, magnesium, copper, manganese, cobalt, etc. may be present. These may also contain coloured prosthetic group like chlorophyll and hemoglobin.
   - *Glycoproteins or mucoproteins*: These contain carbohydrate or derivative of carbohydrate as prosthetic group, e.g. mucins protein of mucus.
   - *Phosphoproteins*: Prosthetic group is phosphoric acid, e.g. caseinogens protein of milk.
   - *Lipoproteins*: Prosthetic group is lecithin, kephalin, etc. e.g. peptone, proteoses, etc.
   - *Metalloproteins*: These are heavy-metal protein complexes, e.g. calcium caseinate.

iii. ***Derived proteins***: These are degradation products by the reaction of acids, alkalis or enzymes on proteins.

Physical properties

These properties give primary idea about identification of a particular protein which can be confirmed by various other specific tests.

Step 1

Solubility test: Solubility of proteins depends upon electric charge of molecule and pH of solution. Proteins show colloidal properties in water and some proteins are completely soluble in water.

1. Appearance of solution	*Turbid* e.g. albumin, globulin, casein		*Clear* e.g. gelatin, peptone
2. Colour of solution	*Opalescent* e.g. albumin, casein	*Faint yellow* e.g. peptone	*Faint brown* e.g. gelatin

Step 2

Smell test

1. *General test*: Some proteins possess characteristic smell so can be identified by smell.

Egg like smell	*Milk like smell*	*Meat like smell*
e.g. albumin	e.g. casein	e.g. peptone, gelatin

2. *Heat test*: Proteins when heated in porcelain dish, protein charts and produces characteristic odour of burning flesh.

3. *Nitrogen test*: All proteins contain nitrogen. So, on heating with soda lime (CaO + NaOH) in a test tube, proteins produce ammonia vapours which can be identified by its odour.

Step 3

Litmus test: Proteins possess free amino (basic) and carboxyl (acidic) groups, so proteins are amphoteric in nature and due to this nature proteins can be combined with acids and bases and proteins also act as buffers.

Neutral to litmus	*Acidic to litmus*	*Alkaline to litmus*
e.g. albumin, gelatin	e.g. peptones	e.g. casein, metaproteins

Step 4

Hydrolysis test: All proteins molecules, after hydrolysis, produce its constituent amino acid, metaprotein, proteoses and peptones as intermediary products.

Precipitation properties

Proteins possess minimum solubility at isoelectric point (due to change in pH, at which amino acids do not migrate towards any electric field), concentrated salt solution and solvents like alcohol which depress ionization, also reduce solubility and cause precipitation. Complex anions in acidic solutions (e.g. trichloroacetic acid, sulphosalicylic acid which reacts with basic group) and cations in alkaline solutions (e.g. heavy metals like Hg^{++},Fe^{++} which reacts with acidic group) also precipitates proteins.

Step 1

Heat coagulation test: All proteins, on heating in the presence of acetic acid, coagulate and appear as insoluble mass.

Step 2

Precipitation by alcohol: All proteins precipitate when excess of alcohol is added to acidified solution of proteins.

Step 3

Precipitation by mineral acids: All proteins precipitate when solution of protein is carefully added to conc. nitric acid by sides of test tube containing nitric acid. A white ring of ppt. is formed at junction of two liquids.

Step 4

Precipitation by heavy metals: All proteins precipitate when solution of mercuric chloride or copper sulphate or ferric chloride or basic lead acetate is added drop by drop to the protein solution.

Step 5

Precipitation by neutral salts: All proteins precipitate when solution of protein is saturated by adding crystals of magnesium sulphate salt. A white ppt. of protein is obtained.

Step 6

Precipitation by alkaloidal reagent: Alkaloidal reagent is a term applied to some complex organic acides used to precipitate alkaloid. These agents are also used to precipitate protein solution.

By adding ferrocyanide sol. (saturated sol.)	White ppt. formed
By adding picric acid sol. (10% sol.)	Yellow ppt. formed
By adding trichloroacetic acid (20% sol.)	White ppt. formed
By adding sulphosalicylic acid (10% sol.)	White ppt. formed
By adding tannic acid	Brownish ppt. formed

Colour reaction properties

Proteins give colour reactions due to presence of some constituent, radical or functional group, so all proteins may not give all colour reaction positive.

Step 1

Ninhydrin test: All proteins, protein derivatives and amino acids give positive result to this test due to presence of free amino and a free carboxylic group. The blue coloured complex is produced by the reaction of two molecules of ninhydrin and ammonia and ammonia is librated by oxidation of amino acids.

Reagent: 0.1% ninhydrin in buffer at pH 7.

Step 2

Biuret test: All proteins give positive result to this test due to presence of two peptide linkage (-CO-NH-) in which a complex is formed by reactions of Cu^{++} with –CO and –NH of peptide linkage in alkaline solution. This test confirms presence of protein. To the sample solution, add equal amount of 10% NaOH solution, to this mixture add 2-3 drops of 1% $CuSO_4$.

Violet or purple colour	*Rosy pink colour*
Protein present	Peptones present

Step 3

Xanthoproteic test: Proteins which contain benzene nucleus in their amino acid residue give positive result to this test (yellow–orange colour produced), e.g. phenylalaline, tyrosine and tryptophane, etc.

Reagents (a) Conc. HNO_3
(b) Strong ammonia

Step 4

Molisch's test: Proteins which contain suger in their molecule give positive result to this test, e.g. serum igG, ovalbumin and lactalbumin, etc.

Molish's reagent: 5% α napthol in 95% ethanol.

Step 5

Millon's test: Proteins which contain amino acid tyrosine in their molecule give positive result to this test, e.g. albumin, globuline, casein, peptone, etc. In this test mercuric sulphate of the reagent reacts with proteins to form white precipitates which on heating combines with tyrosine to form red precipitate.

Millon's reagent: 1 part Hg and 2 part conc. HNO_3 (W/V).

Specific tests for peptone

Proteins give colour reactions due to presence of some constituent, radical or functional group, so all proteins may not give all colour reaction positive. Larger molecule of peptone are called proteose.

Step 1

Aldehyde test: Proteins which contain amino acid tryptophan in their molecule give positive result to this test, e.g. peptone, etc. In this test mercuric sulphate of the reagent reacts with proteins to form white precipitates which on condensation with formaldehyde in presence of sulphuric acid form a violet coloured compound with amino acid tryptophan.

Reagents
1. Formalin—40%
2. Mercuric sulphate sol.
3. Conc. H_2SO_4

Step 2

Sulphur test: Proteins which contain sulphur as structural part of amino acid (like cryteine and cystine) give positive result to this test, e.g. peptone, etc. In this test, sulphur from amino acid precipitated as black/brown ppt. of lead sulphide when lead acetate is added to the sample.

Reagents
1. Lead acetate 5% W/V
2. NaOH sol. —1N

Specific tests for gelatin

Proteins give colour reactions due to presence of some constituent, radical or functional group, so all proteins may not give all colour reaction positive.

Step 1

Arginine test or sakaguchi reaction: Proteins which contain amino acid arginine give positive result to this test, e.g. gelatin, etc. In this test, guanidine group of amino acid arginine reacts with ά-naphthol in presence of sodium hypobromite (NaOBr), produces red orange condensate.

Reagents
1. NaOH — 10%
2. α-naphthol — 1%
3. NaOBr — Can be prepared by adding bromine water to 10% NaOH sol. till yellow colour is obtained.

Stepwise Details for Identification of given Sample of Protein

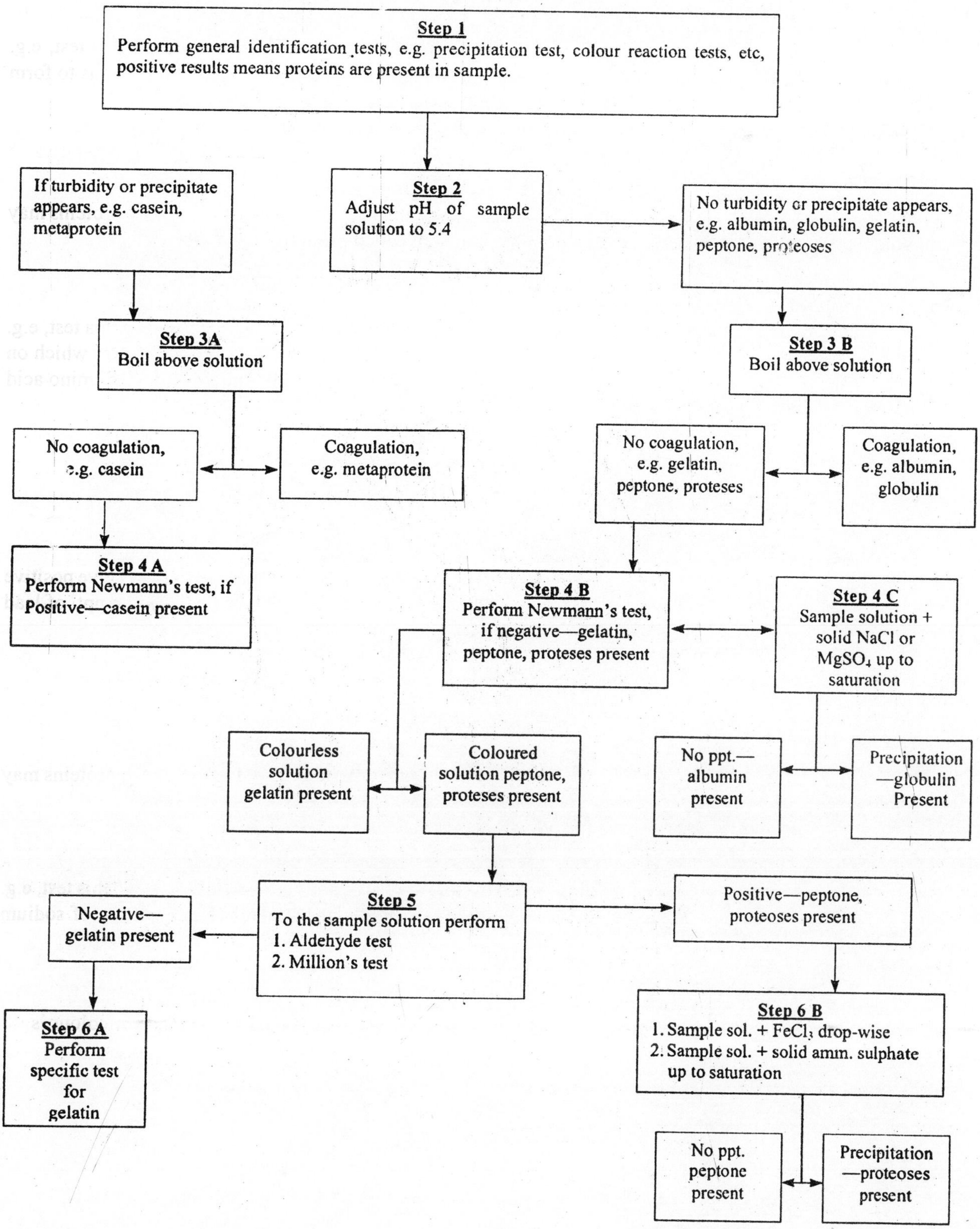

Experiment 15

OBJECT

To identify the given sample of protein (albumin).

S. no.	Test	Observation	Inference
A.	**Physical test**		
1.	Colour		
2.	Smell		
3.	Solubility test		
B.	**Chemical test**		
1.	***Molisch's test***: To the sample solution add 2 drops of 1-naphthol sol., add conc. sulphuric acid.		
2.	***Biuret test***: To the sample solution, add 1% $CuSO_4$ sol. and add excess NaOH.		
3.	***Nitrogen test***: To the dry sample, add 3 times mixture of powder NaOH + CaO, heat and place a glass rod, previously dipped in HCl, over the mouth of test tube.		
4.	***Phosphorus test***: To the sample powder, add 2 ml H_2SO_4 + HNO_3 + excess of amm. molybdate, boil.		
5.	***Sulphur test***: To the protein sample add, 2 ml NaOH, 2 drops of lead sub-acetate.		

S. no.	*Test*	*Observation*	*Inference*
6.	***Rosenhim's test:*** To the sample, add dil. HCHO + H_2SO_4 containing traces of ferric chloride.		
7.	***Xanthoproteic test:*** To the solution, add conc. nitric acid and heat, after cooling add conc. ammonia.		
8.	***Heat coagulation test:*** To the dil. sample sol. add 2% acetaldehyde and heat.		

Conclusion

The given sample is ....

Remarks

1. Albumin is simple protein.
2. Albumins are soluble in water and dilute salt solution.
3. Coagulation temperature of albumins from different sources, differs and normally coagulation starts at 75° C.

Experiment 16

OBJECT

To identify the given sample of protein (casein).

S. no.	*Test*	*Observation*	*Inference*
A.	**Physical test**		
1.	Colour		
2.	Smell		
3.	Solubility test		
B.	**Chemical test**		
1.	***Molisch's test***: To the sample solution add 2 drops of 1-naphthol sol., add conc. sulphuric acid.		
2.	***Biuret test***: To the sample solution add 1% $CuSO_4$ sol., add excess NaOH.		
3.	***Nitrogen test***: To the dry sample, add 3 times mixture of powder NaOH + CaO, heat and place a glass rod, previously dipped in HCl, over the mouth of test tube.		
4.	***Phosphorus test***: To the sample powder, add 2 ml H_2SO_4 + HNO_3 + excess of amm. molybdate, boil.		
5.	***Sulphur test***: To the protein sample add, 2 ml NaOH, 2 drops of lead sub-acetate.		

S. no.	*Test*	*Observation*	*Inference*
6.	***Rosenhim's test***: To the sample added dil. HCHO + H_2SO_4 containing traces of ferric chloride.		
7.	***Xanthoproteic test***: To the solution add nitric acid and heat, after cooling add conc. ammonia.		
8.	***Heat coagulation test***: To the dil. sample sol. add 2% acetaldehyde and heat.		

Conclusion

The given sample is ....

Remarks

1. Casein is milk protein.
2. Casein is a phospho-protein.

Experiment 17

OBJECT

To identify the given sample of protein (gelatin).

S. no.	*Test*	*Observation*	*Inference*
A.	**Physical test**		
1.	Colour		
2.	Smell		
3.	Solubility test		
B.	**Chemical test**		
1.	***Molisch's test***: To the sample solution add 2 drops of 1-naphthol sol., add conc. sulphuric acid.		
2.	***Biuret test***: To the sample solution add 1% $CuSO_4$ sol., add excess NaOH.		
3.	***Nitrogen test***: To the dry sample, add 3 times mixture of powder NaOH + CaO, heat and place a glass rod, previously dipped in HCl, over the mouth of test tube.		
4.	***Phosphorus test***: To the sample powder add 2 ml H_2SO_4 + HNO_3 + excess of amm. molybdate, boil.		
5.	***Sulphur test***: To the protein sample add, 2 ml NaOH, 2 drops of lead sub-acetate.		

S. no.	Test	Observation	Inference
6.	***Rosenhim's test***: To the sample add dil. HCHO + H_2SO_4 containing traces of ferric chloride.		
7.	***Xanthoproteic test***: To the solution add conc. nitric acid and heat, after cooling add conc. ammonia.		
8.	***Heat coagulation test***: To the dil. sample sol. add 2% acetaldehyde and heat.		
9.	***Sakaguchi test:***		

Conclusion

The given sample is ....

Remarks

1. General test for protein positive, possibility of gelatin.
2. At pH 5.4 no turbidity or precipitate, no heat coagulation, possibility of gelatin.
3. Soluble in water and dilute salt solution. Possibility of gelatin.
4. Rosenheim's test negative, so given sample is gelatin.
5. Biuret test is positive, so given sample is gelatin.
6. Performed Argining test or Sakaguchi rèaction. Sample is gelatin.

Experiment 18

OBJECT

To identify the given sample of protein (peptone).

S. no.	*Test*	*Observation*	*Inference*
A.	**Physical test**		
1.	Colour		
2.	Smell		
3.	Solubility test		
B.	**Chemical test**		
1.	***Molisch's test*:** To the sample solution add 2 drops of 1-naphthol sol., add conc. sulphuric acid.		
2.	***Biuret test*:** To the sample solution add 1% $CuSO_4$ sol., add excess NaOH.		
3.	***Nitrogen test*:** To the dry sample, add 3 times mixture of powder NaOH + CaO, heat and place a glass rod, previously dipped in HCl, over the mouth of test tube.		
4.	***Phosphorus test*:** To the sample powder add 2 ml H_2SO_4 + HNO_3 + excess of amm. molybdate, boil.		
5.	***Sulphur test*:** To the protein sample add, 2 ml NaOH, 2 drops of lead sub-acetate.		

S. no.	*Test*	*Observation*	*Inference*
6.	***Rosenhim's test***: To the sample add dil. HCHO + H_2SO_4 containing traces of ferric chloride.		
7.	***Xanthoproteic test***: To the solution add conc. nitric acid and heat, after cooling add conc. ammonia.		
8.	***Heat coagulation test***: To the dil. sample sol. add 2% acetaldehyde and heat.		
9.	To dilute sample sol., add 3-4 drop of mercuric nitrate.		

Conclusion

The given sample is ....

Remarks

1. General test for protein positive, possibility of peptone.
2. At pH 5.4 no turbidity or precipitate, no heat coagulation, possibility of peptone.
3. Soluble in water and dilute salt solution. Possibility of peptone.
4. Aldehyde test and sulphur test positive, so given sample is peptone.
5. Newmann's test is negative, so given sample may be peptone.
6. Performed Argining test or Sakaguchi reaction (negative). Sample is peptone.
7. Peptone reacts with mercuric nitrate sol. to give white ppts. which dissolve in saturated sol. of NaCl.

Experiment 19

OBJECT

To identify the given sample of protein.

S. no.	*Test*	*Observation*	*Inference*
A.	**Physical test**		
1.	Colour		
2.	Smell		
3.	Solubility test		
B.	**Chemical test**		
1.	***Molisch's test*:** To the sample solution add 2 drops of 1-naphthol sol., add conc. sulphuric acid.		
2.	***Biuret test*:** To the sample solution add 1% $CuSO_4$ sol., add excess NaOH.		
3.	***Nitrogen test*:** To the dry sample, add 3 times mixture of powder NaOH + CaO, heat and place a glass rod, previously dipped in HCl, over the mouth of test tube.		
4.	***Phosphorus test*:** To the sample powder add 2 ml H_2SO_4 + HNO_3 + excess of amm. molybdate, boil.		
5.	***Sulphur test*:** To the protein sample add, 2 ml NaOH, 2 drops of lead sub-acetate.		

S. no.	*Test*	*Observation*	*Inference*
6.	***Rosenhim's test***: To the sample add dil. HCHO + H_2SO_4 containing traces of ferric chloride.		
7.	***Xanthoproteic test***: To the solution add conc. nitric acid and heat, after cooling add conc. ammonia.		
8.	***Heat coagulation test***: To the dil. sample sol. add 2% acetaldehyde and heat.		

Conclusion

The given sample is ....

Remarks

Experiment 20

OBJECT

To identify the given sample of protein.

S. no.	*Test*	*Observation*	*Inference*
A.	**Physical test**		
1.	Colour		
2.	Smell		
3.	Solubility test		
B.	**Chemical test**		
1.	***Molisch's test***: To the sample solution add 2 drops of 1-naphthol sol., add conc. sulphuric acid.		
2.	***Biuret test***: To the sample solution add 1% $CuSO_4$ sol., add excess NaOH.		
3.	***Nitrogen test***: To the dry sample, add 3 times mixture of powder NaOH + CaO, heat and place a glass rod, previously dipped in HCl, over the mouth of test tube.		
4.	***Phosphorus test***: To the sample powder add 2 ml H_2SO_4 + HNO_3 + excess of amm. molybdate, boil.		
5.	***Sulphur test***: To the protein sample add, 2 ml NaOH, 2 drops of lead sub-acetate.		

S. no.	*Te'*	*Observation*	*Inference*
6.	***Rosenhim's test*:** To the sample add dil. HCHO + H_2SO_4 containing traces of ferric chloride.		
7.	***Xanthoproteic test*:** To the solution add conc. nitric acid and heat, after cooling add conc. ammonia.		
8.	***Heat coagulation test*:** To the dil. sample sol. add 2% acetaldehyde and heat.		

Conclusion

The given sample is ....

Remarks

4

Urine Analysis

Kidney plays an important role in urine formation which involves glomerular filtration, tubular reabsorption and tubular secretion. Urine composition is effected by nutritional status, metabolic process and the physiology of kidney.

Collection of Urine

It should be collected in dry, clean container. It is examined freshly. A morning specimen is taken for renal diseases. For diabetes mellitus sample is collected after two hours of intake of food.

Physical properties

The colour of urine is due to presence of pigment urochrome (a breakdown product of hemoglobin), transparent to pale yellow or dark amber coloured. The characteristic aromatic odour of urine is produced due to decomposition of urea to ammonia. Average amount of urine formed in a day is about 1500 ml, which depends upon intake of water and weather temperature. pH range of fresh urine is 6 to 8.6, specific gravity range 1.010 to 1.025 in normal condition.

Preservation

Urine may be preserve by adding two percent toluene or formaline or thymol.

Composition

Specific gravity	1.010 – 1.025
pH	6 – 8.6 (Average pH 6)
Inorganic constituents per 24 hours	
Iron	0.06 – 0.1 mg
Chloride	4 – 10 gm on usual diet
Sodium	4 gm on usual diet
Sulphur	2 gm
Phosphate	0.8 – 0.3 gm on usual diet
Calcium	< 150 mg
Organic constituents per 24 hours	
Urea	15 – 30 gm
Creatinine	1 – 1.8 gm
Ammonium	0.3 – 1 gm
Uric acid	0.3 – 0.6 gm
Albumin	0 – 0.1 gm
Amylase (diastase)	40 – 260 units per hour
Quantity per day	½ – 1.5 litre

Classification

- ***Physiological or normal urine***: If urine contains only waste product and it does not contain any product required by the body, called physiological or normal urine.
- ***Pathological or abnormal urine***: Due to some physiological disorders if urine contains substances that are essential to the body, e.g. sugar, ketone body, bile salts and albumin, etc. These abnormal constituents of urine indicate some disease or renal disorder.

Abnormal constituent	*Condition*	*Cause*
Sugar (glucose)	Glycosuria	Due to diabetes mellitus
Ketone bodies	Ketosis	Due to diabetes mellitus/pregnancy/anesthesia, etc.
Protein	Proteinuria	Due to excesses physical activity/high protein diet/ pregnancy/nephritis and nephrosis.
Albumin	Albuminuria	Due to nephritis
Bile pigments and salts (Sod. glycocholate and sod. tarocholate are salts and bilirubin and biliveridine are pigments.		Due to jaundice
Pus cells	Pyuria	Due to infection in urine balder/ urethra or kidney.
Blood or blood cells	Haematuria	Due to tuberculosis, cancer/ jaundice/ renal stone/ inflammation of renal organs/ malaria/ typhoid/ poison/ burn, etc.
Haemoglobin	Haemoglobinurea	
Excess urea	Uremia	Due to bacterial infection.

Examination of urine

It contains the following tests.

1. Physical test
2. Chemical test
3. Microscopic

Physical Test

Appearance

Normal urine is clear. The cloudy urine is indicative of the presence of pus, RBC's or bacteria.

1. ***Colour***: The colour of normal urine is straw (pale yellow).
   (i) *Milky*: Chyluria.
   (ii) *Cloudy*: Phosphate, urates.
   (iii) *Orange*: Concentrated urine, fever, urobilin.
   (iv) *Red*: Haematuria, pyridium.
   (v) *Green*: Biliverdin, phenol poisoning.
   (vi) *Dark brown*: Myoglobin, acute febrile condition.
2. ***Reaction*** : Average pH – 6.

It can be measured by litmus paper or by pH metre. Acidic urine is seen in ketosis, metabolic acidosis and UTI, where as alkaline urine is found in systemic alkalosis, UTI, alkalinization and therapy like sulfonamides, streptomycin, etc.

3. ***Specific gravity***: It can be measured by urinometre or refractometre. High specific gravity is seen in glycosuria, acute nephritis, albuminuria, etc. Whereas low specific gravity (less than 1.010) is found in excessive water intake, chronic nephritis and diabetes insipidus.

4. ***Urinary volume***: (0.5 to 1.5 ltr. per day)

Polyuria: Urine output is more than 2 litres.
Oliguria: Urine excretion is less than 0.5 litre.
Anuria: Stopage of urination.

5. ***Odour***: Normal urine is aromatic in smell but its smell turms ammonical on standing. Pathologically, it is sweetish in ketosis, putrid in cystitis and faecal in fistula.

Chemical Test

Normal constituents

(i) ***Chloride***: The urine (2 ml) is acidified with dilute HNO_3 (2 to 3 drops) and $AgNO_3$ solution (1 ml) is added. A white precipitate is positive for chloride.

(ii) ***Sulphate***: The urine (2 ml) is acidified with dilute HCl (2 to 3 drops) and barium chloride solution is added. A white precipitate shows the presence of sulphate in urine.

(iii) ***Phosphate***: The urine (2 ml) is acidified with dilute HNO_3 and dilute H_2SO_4 (2 to 3 drops of each). Excess of ammonium molybdate is added. A yellow precipitate shows the presence of phosphate.

(iv) ***Urea***

(a) A small quantity of urine is taken in dry test tube, 1 ml of mercuric nitrate solution is added. A white precipitate is obtained showing the presence of urea.

(b) A small quantity of urine is taken in a dry test tube, add 1 ml of oxime solution and 1 ml of acid solution. Mix properly and place the test tube in boiling water bath for ten minutes. Cool it. A specific pink colour complex is obtained showing the presence of urea in urine.

(v) ***Ammonium salt***: Take specific quantity (2 ml) of urine into a test tube. Add 1 to 2 drops of phenolphthalein and sodium carbonate solution drop by drop till pink colour is developed. A glass rod dipped with phenolphthalein is kept (not to be touched) near the mouth of the test tube. The glass rod containing phenolphthalein layer turns pink due to release of ammonia gas.

(vi) ***Creatinine***: It reacts with alkaline picrate to form red coloured complex. Take 0.5 ml of urine. Add 3 ml of saturated solution of picric acid and 1 ml of 10 percent W/V sodium hydroxide solution. Mix well and keep at room temperature for 10 minutes. A deep reddish orange colour is formed.

(vii) ***Uric acid***

(a) *Schiff's test*: Take a filter paper moistened with $AgNO_3$ solution. Put 1 to 2 drops of alkaline urine (make alkaline urine by adding sodium carbonate solution). A black precipitate of metallic silver is obtained on the paper if uric acid is present.

(b) *Phosphotungstate reagent*: Take small quantity of urine and adjust the urine pH to 10 with solid sodium carbonate. To it add 2 ml phosphotungstate reagent and make it alkaline with saturated sodium carbonate solution. A blue colour is indicative of the presence of uric acid.

Reagents

Oxime solution

Diacetyl monoxine	1 gm
Thiosemicarbazide	0.2 gm
Sodium chloride	9 gm

Dissolve the ingredients and dilute the solution to make up to 1000 ml with distilled water. Stability of this solution is 21 days.

Acid solution

Conc. H_2SO_4	60 ml
Phosphoric acid 85%	10 ml
Ferric chloride	0.1 gm

Take 800 ml of distilled water in 1 litre volumetric flask. Add the above ingredients carefully and make-up the volume to 1000 ml with distilled water. Stability is 60 days.

Phosphotungstic acid reagent

Take 350 ml of distilled water into a RB flask. Add 50 gm of sodium tungstate and 32 ml of 82% ortho-phosphoric acid. Put some glass beads into RB flask. Reflex the mixture for a period of two hours. Take out the flask from the condenser attachment and add a drop of bromine. Boil for a few minutes. Then cool and dilute to 1000 ml in a graduated cylinder. To increase the stability and sensitivity of the reagent lithium sulphate (32 gm) is added to above reagent.

Experiment 21

OBJECT

To carry out physical examination of given sample of urine.

Date: ——————————.
Name of the patient/individual: ——————————.
Age: ——————————.
Sex: ——————————.
Referred by: ——————————.

Physical Test

1. Colour :
   Normal : Straw or pale yellow
   Abnormal : Milky/cloudy/orange/red/green/dark brown
2. Appearance : Clear/turbid/hazy
3. Reaction : Acidic/alkaline
4. Specific gravity : (1.010 to 1.025)
5. Urinary volume : 0.5 to 1.5 litre in 24 hours
6. Odour : Aromatic/putrid/faecal/pungent

Result

Normal/abnormal.

Experiment 22

OBJECT

To analyze the given sample of urine for its normal inorganic constitutions.

Chemical Test

S. no.	*Test*	*Observation*	*Inference*
1.	Chloride		
2.	Sulphate		
3.	Phosphate		
4.	Ammonium salt		

Result

Experiment 23

OBJECT

To analyze the given sample of urine for its normal organic constitutions.

Chemical Test

S.no.	Test	Observation	Inference
1.	Test for urea		
	(a) Mercuric nitrate solution		
	(b) Oxime reagent		
2.	Creatinine (Alkaline picrate test)		
3.	Uric acid		
	(a) Schiff's test		
	(b) Phosphate tungstate reagent test		

Result

CHEMICAL TEST OF URINE

Abnormal Constituents

1. Test for protein (Albumin)

Normal value: Negative or trace (2 – 8 mg per dl).

(a) *Acetic acid test*: Fill ¾ of a test tube with fresh urine, boil upper part of the urine for 2 minutes. A turbidity may be produced due to phosphates, carbonates or albumin. A few drops of 10% acetic acid is added. The development of turbidity indicates the presence of albumin in urine.

Interpretation:

No turbidity	:	Negative
Cloudiness	:	+ (Positive)
Granular cloudiness	:	++ (Positive)
Dense opaque cloud	:	+++ (Positive)
Very thick curdy ppt.	:	++++ (Positive)

(b) *Sulphosalicylic acid test*: Take specific amount of urine and add a few drops of sulphosalicylic acid (20%). The presence of turbidity indicates the albumin after boiling a few minutes.
The presence of tolbutamide, penicillin, etc. may give false positive test.
If turbidity disappears on heating and reappear of cooling, it is Bence Jones protein.

(c) *Paper strip*: Many manufacturers provide strip for rapid diagnostics, i.e. uristix, multistix (Miles India Ltd.)

Clinical significance

Proteinuria: Protein in urine. It is seen in fever, stress, hypertension, UTI, congestive heart failure, glomerular nephritis, myeloma, nephrotic syndrome, trauma, leukemia, hyperthyroidism, etc.
A false positive test may be found in the following conditions.
Alkaline urine, drug like acetazolamide, thymol, arsenic, etc.

2. Test for glucose

Normal value: Negative.

(a) *Benedict's qualitative test*: To 5 ml of Benedict's reagent, add 0.5 ml of urine. Heat to boiling over a flame for two minutes. Observe as follow:

Blue to green	:	Negative
Yellowish green	:	+ (< 0.5% glucose)
Greenish yellow	:	++ (0.5 – 1 % glucose)
Yellow	:	+++ (1 – 2 % glucose)
Orange to brick red	:	++++ (> 2 % glucose)

(b) *Fehling's test*: To 2 ml of urine, add 2ml of Fehling's reagents (Fehling's reagent A and B in equal volume). Mix and boil the solution. Observe colour change green, yellow to brick red indicates the presence of glucose (reducing sugar) in urine.

(c) *Paper strip*: It is available for rapid test based on glucose oxidase method, i.e. diastix (Miles India Ltd.), glucostripes (Hi tech).

Clinical significance

Glycosuria: Presence of glucose in urine. Glycosuria is seen in diabetes mellitus, Cushing's syndrome, hyperthyroidism, pheochromocytoma, pancreatic disease, severe burns, sepsis, cardiac shock, etc. Drugs like corticosteroids, thiazides, oral contraceptives, etc. Also cause glycosuria.

3. Ketone bodies

Normal value: Negative.

Ketone bodies include acetone 2%, aceto-acetic acid (20%) and ß hydroxyl butyric acid (78%). Ketone bodies are produced by incomplete fat metabolism and their presence is indicative of acidosis.

(a) *Rothera's test*: 5 ml of urine is saturated with solid ammonium sulphate and a few crystals of sodium nitroprusside are added. Mix thoroughly, liquid ammonia is added from the side of the test tube, formation of a purple ring at the junction shows a positive test.

(b) *Paper strip*: Multistix (Miles India Ltd.), Keto-Diastix, etc. These strips contain sodium nitroprusside, amino acetic acid and di-sodium phosphate. A purple colour is develop indicating the positive test.

Clinical significance

Ketonuria: Ketone bodies in urine.

Causes of ketonuria

1. *Diabetic mellitus*: Uncontrolled ketoacidosis may give rise to coma.
2. *Non-diabetic ketonuria*: It occurs in fever, anorexia, starvation and prolonged vomiting.

Drugs may cause false positive test, i.e. lavodopa, metformin, ether, insulin, and phenformin.

4. Bile pigments

Normal value: < 0.02 mg %

(a) *Foam test:* 5 ml of urine in a test tube is shaken. Bile pigments produce a yellowish foam. This test in not accurate as protein can also form foam.

(b) *Gmelin's test:* Take 3 ml of fuming nitric acid in a test tube and add 3 ml of urine at the side of the test tube gently. A green or blue ring indicates bilirubin.

Clinical significance

Increase amount of bilirubin in urine is termed as hyper bilirubinuria. It is seen in chronic hepatocellular damage and obstruction of bile duct.

5. Bile salt

Hays test: Fill the test tube with urine sample. Sprinkle powdered sulphur over the surface. If bile salts are present the sulphur particles will sink.

Clinical significance

In obstructive jaundice: Bile salts along with bilirubin are present.

6. Blood

(a) *Benzidine test:* 2 ml of glacial acetic acid is saturated with benzidine. Add 1 ml of fresh hydrogen peroxide and 2 ml of urine. Development of blue or green colour is the indicative of blood present in urine.

(b) *Paper strip*: Blood acts with the peroxide-ortho-toluidine reagent to form blue colour. Hemastix is available.

Clinical significance

Haematuria: Blood in urine is seen in disorder of kidney and genito-urinary tract. Sulphonamides, dicoumarol, etc. cause drug induced haematuria.

Experiment 24

OBJECT

To analyze the given sample of urine for its abnormal constitutions.

Chemical Test

S. no.	*Test*	*Observation*	*Inference*
1.	Test for albumin (a) Acetic acid test (b) Sulpho-salicylic acid test		
2.	Glucose (a) Benedict's test (b) Fehling's test		
3.	Blood Benzidine test		

Result

Experiment 25

OBJECT

To analyze the given sample of urine for its abnormal constitutions.

Chemical Test

S. no.	*Test*	*Observation*	*Inference*
1.	Ketone bodies Rothera's test		
2.	Bile pigments (a) Foam test		
	(b) Gmelin's test		
3.	Bile salt Hays test		

Result

Experiment 26

OBJECT

To report diastase content in urine/serum/plasma.

Iodometric Method

Principle

Diastase is amylolytic enzyme, acts on starch to form maltose. Diastase activity is defined as number of mg of starch substrate, hydrolysed by it under standard condition. It is measured by the loss of blue colour in the test after the addition of iodine compared with a control in which enzymatic hydrolysis is prevented. One unit of diastase will hydrolyse 5 mg of starch to the point where no blue colour is given with iodine in 15 minutes at 37° C.

$$\text{Diastase activity in units per dl} = \frac{\text{Absorbance of control} - \text{Absorbance of test}}{\text{Absorbance of control}} \times 800$$

The factor of 800 is calculated as follow.

$$\frac{100}{0.1} \times \frac{2}{5} \times \frac{15}{7.5}$$

0.1	:	Amount of serum/plasma
2	:	2 mg of starch substrate is taken
5	:	5 mg of starch under standard condition
15	:	15 minutes of incubation at 37° C
7.5	:	7.5 minutes of incubation of test solution at 37° C
1 dl	=	100 ml.

Reagents

1. *Buffered starch substrate (pH 7)*: Dissolve 22.6 gm reagent grade anhydrous disodium hydrogen phosphate (Na_2HPO_4) and 12.6 gm. AR grade potassium dihydrogen phosphate (KH_2PO_4) in 500 ml of 0.9% W/V sodium chloride solution. Boil the above solution and add 0.4 gm soluble starch in 10 ml of 0.9% sodium chloride solution. Cool and add 5 ml of 37% formaldyhyde. Adjust the volume up to 1 litre with 0.9% sodium chloride solution.
2. *0.1 N iodine solution*: Dissolve 3.567 gm of potassium iodate in approximately 800 ml distilled water. Add 9 ml conc. HCl and dilute to 1 litre. Keep in a brown bottle.
3. *Working 0.1 N iodine solution*: Dilute 50 ml of stock iodone solution up to 500 ml with distilled water.

Procedure

Take two conical flasks and is marked T (test) and C (control). Add 5 ml of buffered starch substrate in to each flask. Warm the test flask for 5 minutes in 37° C at water bath. Add 0.1 ml of fresh sample (serum/plasma/urine). Mix well and incubate the test flask exactly 7.5 minutes in 37° C at water bath. Add 5 ml of working iodine solution (0.01 N) to both flasks. Adjust the volume of both flask to 50 ml with distilled water of mix well. Note the absorbance of both test and control at 660 nm, setting zero absorbance with water.

Result

Normal value (serum/plasma)	:	60–160 units/dl
Normal value (urine)	:	40–260 units/hour

Clinical significance

It is estimated in diagnosis of diseases of pancreas. Increase in diastase activity is observed in case of mumps, cholicystitis and salivary glands lesions.

Experiment 27

OBJECT

Quantitative determination of glucose in urine by *o*-toluidine method.

Reagents

Glucose kit (J. Mitra and Co. Ltd.)

This kit contains glucose reagent (*o*-toluidine) and standard glucose solution (100 mg per dl).

Principle

O-toluidine in hot acetic acid reacts with glucose to form blue–green colour complex glucosamine. The intensity of colour is directly proportional to the concentration of glucose.

Procedure

Three test tubes are taken labeled as B (blank), S (standard) and T (test).

S. no.	*Reagent*	*Blank*	*Standard*	*Test*
1.	Glucose reagent	3 ml	3 ml	3 ml
2.	Distilled water	50 μl	—	—
3.	Glucose standard	—	50 μl	—
4.	Sample urine	—	—	50 μl

Mix well and heat the test and standard labeled test tubes into boiling water bath (100° C) for exactly 9 minutes. Cool the both test tubes at room temperature or by placing in cold water. Measure absorbance (optical densities) of S and T test tubes against blank adjusted to zero. The analyzer must be set at 620 ± 20 nm.

Calculation

$$\text{Glucose conc. per dl} = \frac{\text{OD of test sample}}{\text{OD of standard}} \times 100$$

$$\text{OD} = \text{Optical density}$$

Result

.... mg per dl.

Diagnostic significance

Glucose in urine or blood is reported in diabetes mellitus, hyper activity of pituitary, thyroid and adrenal glands. Hypoglycemia is observed in case of insulin overdose, hypopituatrism, hypoadrenalism, etc.

Experiment 28

OBJECT

Quantitative determination of urea in urine.

Reagents

Urea kit (J. Mitra and Co, Ltd.)
This kit contains the following reagents.
Urea colour reagent A (oxime solution).
Urea colour reagent B (ferric salt solution).
Urea acid reagent C.
Urea standard 40 mg per dl.

Principle

Diacetyl monoxime in acidic medium at 100° C reacts with urea to form pink coloured complex. The presence of ferric ions increase the sensitivity of the colour. The intensity of the colour is directly proportional to the concentration of urea into test sample. The absorbance (optical density) is measured colorimetrically at 520 nm.

Procedure

The three dry and cleaned test tubes are taken and marked as B (blank), S (standard) and T (test).

S. no.	*Reagent*	*Blank*	*Standard*	*Test*
1.	Urea colour reagent A (oxime solution)	1.5 ml	1.5 ml	1.5 ml
2.	Urea colour reagent B (ferric salt solution)	1.5 ml	1.5 ml	1.5 ml
3.	Urea acid reagent C	2 ml	2 ml	2 ml
4.	Distilled water	50 µl	—	—
5.	Urea standard 40 mg/dl	—	50 µl	—
6.	Sample (urine/serum/plasma)	—	—	50 µl

Add the reagents as above in all three test tubes. Mix well and incubate all test tubes in boiling water bath for exactly 10 minutes. Remove all the three test tubes from water and measure absorbance of S and T tubes at 520 nm against blank adjusted to zero by analyser.

Urine sample must be diluted ten times with distilled water and multiply the final reading by 10.

Calculation

$$\text{Concentration of urea in mg/dl} = \frac{\text{OD of test sample}}{\text{OD of standard}} \times 40 \times D$$

Where D is dilution factor of urine sample.
Normal range: 25 – 40 gm/24 hours.

Result

…………..……………..

Diagnostic significance

Increased levels: Acute glomerulonephritis, fevers, diabetic coma, dehydration and shock.

Decreased level: Viral hepatitis.

Experiment 29

OBJECT

Quantitative determination of creatinine in urine.

Reagents

Creatinine kit (J. Mitra and Co. Ltd.)
This kit contains the following reagents.
Creatinine reagent A (saturated picric acid solution).
Alkaline reagent.
Creatinine standard 150 mg/dl (stock solution).

Principle

Creatinine reacts with alkaline picrate to form red coloured complex. The optical density of red colour is proportional to the amount of creatinine in the sample which is measured at 520 ± 15 nm colorimetrically.

Creatinine + picric acid ⟶ orange coloured complex.

Procedure

Creatinine determination in urine is usually carried out on a 24 hours urine sample. Thymol is used as preservative. The urine sample (1 ml) is diluted to 25 ml with distilled water.

Preparation of working standard solution: Dilute 0.1 ml of stock standard solution to 10 ml with distilled water.

Diproteinization of test sample

Sample/reagent	*Quantity*
Diluted urine/serum	1 ml
Distilled water	1 ml
Creatinine reagent A	6 ml

Mix well and put in boiling water bath for 1 minute. Cool and centrifuge for 5 minutes. Take three test tubes marked as B (blank), S (standard) and T (tests).

S. no.	*Reagent*	*Blank*	*Standard*	*Test*
1.	Supernatant of the above	—	—	4 ml
2.	Working standard	—	1 ml	—
3.	Distilled water	1 ml	—	—
4.	Creatinine reagent A	3 ml	3 ml	—
5.	Alkali reagent	1 ml	1 ml	1 ml

Mix well and allow to stand at room temperature for 20 minutes. Measure the absorbance of blank, standard, and test against distilled water adjusted to zero at 520 nm.

Calculation

$$\text{Urine creatinine in gm/litre} = \frac{\text{OD of test sample} - \text{OD of blank}}{\text{OD of standard} - \text{OD of blank}} \times 0.75 = A$$

Urine creatinine gm/24 hours = A × 24
Urine volume collected in litres.

Result

Normal value
Male : 1.1–2.8 gm/24 hours.
Female : 0.9–1.6 gm/24 hours.

Clinical significance

Increased level: Impaired renal functions.
Decreased level: Muscular dystrophy.

Experiment 30

OBJECT

Quantitative determination of creatine in urine.

Reagents

Creatinine reagent A (saturated picric acid solution).
Alkaline reagent
Creatinine standard 150 mg/dl (stock solution).

Principle

Creatine can be converted to creatinine by autoclaving in presence of acid. The creatinine contents in urine is then estimated by alkaline picrate method.

Urine creatine = 1.16 {creatinine of autoclaved urine sample (T1) – creatinine of non-autoclaved urine sample (T2)}.

Procedure

Take stoppered iodine flask, add 1 ml of ammonium chloride and 1 ml of urine. Autoclave it at 121° C for 20 minutes.

The urine sample 1 ml is diluted to 25 ml with distilled water.

Preparation of working standard solution—Dilute 0.1 ml of stock standard solution to 10 ml with distilled water.

Deproteinization of test samples.

Sample/reagent	Quantity (T1)	Quantity (T2)
Diluted urine/serum	1 ml	1 ml
Distilled water	1 ml	1 ml
Creatinine reagent A	6 ml	6 ml

Mix well and put in boiling water bath for 1 minute. Cool and centrifuge for 5 minutes. Take three test tubes marked as B (blank), S (standard), T_1 (test) and T_2 (test).

S. no.	*Reagent*	*Blank*	*Standard*	*Test (T1)*	*Test (T2)*
1.	Supernatant of the above	—	—	4 ml	4 ml
2.	Working standard	—	1 ml	—	—
3.	Distilled water	1 ml	—	—	—
4.	Creatinine reagent A	3 ml	3 ml	—	—
5.	Alkali reagent	1 ml	1 ml	1 ml	1 ml

Mix well and allow to stand at room temperature for 20 minutes. Measure the absorbance of blank, standard, T1 (autoclaved urine sample) and T2 (non-autoclaved urine sample) against distilled water adjusted to zero at 520 nm colorimetrically.

Calculation

$$\text{Urine creatinine in gm/litre} = \frac{\text{OD of test (T1)} - \text{OD of blank}}{\text{OD of standard} - \text{OD of blank}} \times 0.75 = A$$

$$\text{Urine creatinine in gm/litre} = \frac{\text{OD of test (T2)} - \text{OD of blank}}{\text{OD of standard} - \text{OD of blank}} \times 0.75 = B$$

Urine creatinine in gm/litre in 24 hours (T1) = A × 24.
Urine creatinine in gm/litre in 24 hours (T2) = B × 24.

Urine creatine = 1.16 × (T1–T2).

Result

Normal value: 0–200 mg/24 hours.

5

Clinical Blood Chemistry

Analysis of normal and abnormal constituents of blood is carried out by photocolorimeter (analyzer). So photocolorimeter is the basic requirement in clinical chemistry which is available in various models. Nowadays digital analyzer is available in market which is simple to operate and direct result can be noted. Commercially, available colorimeters have optical density and transmission scales which follow the Beer's and Lambert's laws.

Beer's law

It states that equal thickness of an absorbing material will absorb a constant fraction of the energy incident on it.

Lambert's law

It states that the proportion of light absorbed by an absorbing substance is independent of the intensity of the incident light. The instrument is widely used for clinical laboratories, agricultural analysis, petroleum and water pollution, etc.

Colorimetric analysis is performed for the quantitative determination coloured substance in solution. The general instruments (deflection type) comprises the following parts.

1. *Light source*: Tungsten filament lamp.
2. *Optical system*: It consists of reflector lens.
3. *Filter wheel*: For selecting appropriate wavelength complimentary to the colour of the sample.
4. *Shutter*: It permits light to fall photo cell.
5. *Cuvette*: For placing test tube containing solution being examined.
6. *Photo cell:* For detecting amount of light passing through the solution.
7. *Calibrated micrometre*: For measurement of optical density and percentage transmission.

Selection of filter

Select the filter in that region of the spectrum which gives maximum reading of optical density. In this region the rate of change of optical density is quite sensitive to the rate of change of concentration.

Operation

Make necessary power connection and switch on the instrument. Select the appropriate filter. Set the metre reading on 100% transmission (zero optical density) by using a blank solution in the test tube. It is done by adjusting the concern knob. Then keep the shutter in open position. Insert the standard and test solutions and note the optical densities of the both respectively. Calculate the concentration of test solution as follow.

$$\frac{\text{OD of test}}{\text{OD of standard}} = \frac{\text{Conc. of test}}{\text{Conc. of standard}}$$

$$\text{So conc. of test} = \frac{\text{OD of test}}{\text{OD of standard}} \times \text{conc. of standard}$$

Blood collection

The blood is collected by vein-puncture. Heparin is the most ideal anticoagulant for most of the blood constituents. For glucose oxalate–fluoride mixture is used. All measurements should be performed immediately after collection. For obtaining serum let the blood clot at room temperature. The blood should centrifuge for 10 minutes at 3000 rpm. The serum can be remove by a Pasteur pipette and be stored in a refrigerator at 4 to 6° C until analyzed.

Precautions

1. Centrifuge tube must be balance by placing them in opposite position.
2. Use always dry, clean glass ware.
3. Avoid haemolysis as it imparts RBC contents like potassium, acid phosphatase, etc.
4. Use disposable needle of gauge less than 21 for withdrawal of blood sample.
5. Always mix blood with anticoagulants by gentle inversion about 5 to 10 times.
6. Remove serum immediately after clotting of the blood.
7. The blood specimen should be stored properly.
8. If estimation of the blood constituents are carried out by using readymade reagent kit supplied by various manufactures, i.e. J. Mitra, span, transasia, etc. follow the manufacturer's instructions strictly.

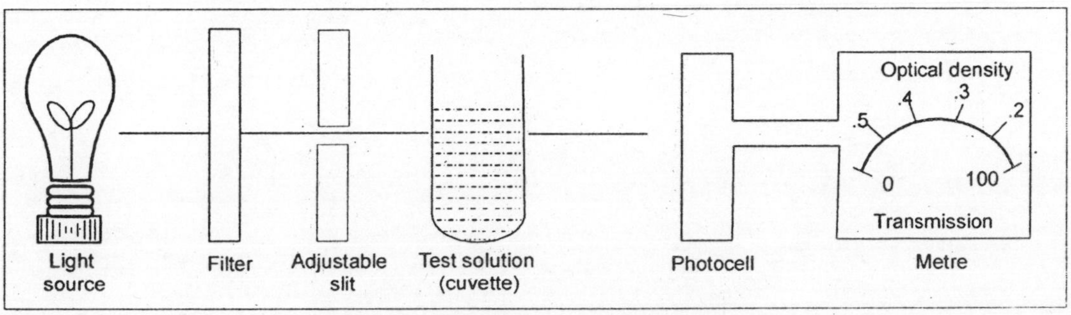

Lab system analyzer (photocolorimeter)

Experiment 31

OBJECT

Quantitative determination of blood sugar (glucose) by *o*-toluidine method.

Reagents

Glucose kit (J. Mitra and Co. Ltd.)
This kit contains glucose reagent (*o*-toluidine) and standard glucose solution (100 mg per dl).

Principle

O-toluidine in hot acetic acid reacts with glucose to form blue–green colour complex glucosamine. The intensity of colour is directly proportional to the concentration of glucose.

Procedure

A. *For serum/plasma without deproteinization*

Three test tubes are taken labeled as B (blank), S (standard), and T (test).

S.no.	*Reagent*	*Blank*	*Standard*	*Test*
1.	Glucose reagent	3 ml	3 ml	3 ml
2.	Distilled water	50 μl	—	—
3.	Glucose standard	—	50 μl	—
4.	Sample plasma/serum	—	—	50 μl

Mix well and heat the test and standard labeled test tubes into boiling water bath (100° C) for exactly 9 minutes. Cool the both test tubes at room temperature or by placing in cold water. Measure absorbance (optical densities) of S and T test tubes against blank adjusted to zero. The analyzer must be set at 620 ± 20 nm.

B. *For whole blood and haemolyzed sample*

In case of whole blood or haemolyzed sample deproteinization by trichloroacetic acid (TCA) is needed. For this take 0.2 ml of sample and add 1.8 ml of 4% TCA solution into centrifuge tube. Mix well and allow to stand for five minutes to precipitate the proteins. Centrifuge for 10 minutes take 3 test tubes mark as B (blank), S (standard), and T (test). Proceed as follow:

S.no.	*Reagent*	*Quantity*		
		B	*S*	*T*
1.	Glucose reagent	3 ml	3 ml	3 ml
2.	Distilled water	0.05 ml	—	—
3.	TCA solution	0.45 ml	0.45 ml	—
4.	Glucose standard	—	0.05 ml	—
5.	Sample supernatant from above	—	—	0.5 ml

Calculation

$$\text{Glucose conc. per dl} = \frac{\text{OD of test sample}}{\text{OD of standard}} \times 100$$

$$\text{OD} = \text{Optical density.}$$

Result

.... mg per dl.

Diagnostic significance

Glucose in urine or blood is reported in diabetes mellitus, hyper activity of pituitary thyroid and adrenal glands. Hypoglycemia is observed in case of insulin overdose, hypopituatrism, hypoadrenalism, etc.

Reagents

1. *O-toluidine*: Dissolve 1.5 gm of thio-urea in 200 ml of glacial acetic acid, add 60 ml of *o*-toludine. Mix and make the volume to 1 litre with glacial acetic acid. Keep in brown bottle. Store at 2–8 °C.
2. *Tri-chloroacetic acid*: 4% W/V.
3. *Standard glucose solution* (100 mg/dl): Dissolve 100 mg in 100 ml of saturated solution of benzoic acid. Store at 2–8 °C.

Experiment 32

OBJECT

Quantitative determination of urea in blood/serum.

Reagents

Urea kit (J. Mitra and Co. Ltd.)
This kit contains the following reagents.
Urea colour reagent A (oxime solution).
Urea colour reagent B (ferric salt solution).
Urea acid reagent C.
Urea standard 40 mg per dl.

Principle

Diacetyl monoxime in acidic medium at 100° C reacts with urea to form pink coloured complex. The presence of ferric ions increase the sensitivity of the colour. The intensity of the colour is directly proportional to the concentration of urea into test sample. The absorbance (optical density) is measured colorimetrically at 520 nm.

Procedure

The three dry and cleaned test tubes are taken and marked as B (blank), S (standard), and T (test).

S. no.	*Reagent*	*Blank*	*Standard*	*Test*
1.	Urea colour reagent A (oxime solution)	1.5 ml	1.5 ml	1.5 ml
2.	Urea colour reagent B (ferric salt solution)	1.5 ml	1.5 ml	1.5 ml
3.	Urea acid reagent C	2 ml	2 ml	2 ml
4.	Distilled water	50 µl	—	—
5.	Urea standard 40 mg/dl	—	50 µl	—
6.	Sample (urine/serum/plasma)	—	—	50 µl

Add the reagents as above in all three test tubes. Mix well and incubate all test tubes in boiling water bath for exactly 10 minutes. Remove all three from water and measure absorbance of S and T tubes at 520 nm against blank adjusted to zero by analyzer.

Calculation

$$\text{Concentration of urea in mg/dl} = \frac{\text{OD of test sample}}{\text{OD of standard}} \times 40$$

Normal range (serum)
Adult : 10 – 46 mg/dl
Children : 10 – 32 mg/dl

Result

....

Diagnostic significance

Increased levels: Acute glomerulonephritis, fevers, diabetic coma, dehydration and shock.

Decreased level: Viral hepatitis.

Reagents

1. Oxime reagent

Diacetyl monoxime	:	1 gm
Thiosemicarbazide	:	0.2 gm
Sodium chloride	:	9 gm

Dissolve the ingredients in sufficient quantity of distilled water in 1 litre volumetric flask. Make up the volume up to 1 litre by distilled water. Store at room temperature.

2. Ferric chloride reagent

0.01 % (store at room temperature).

3. Acid reagent

Conc. H_2SO_4	:	60 ml
Phosphoric acid 85%	:	10 ml

Mix the ingredients in distilled water. Make up the volume up to 1 litre with distilled water. Store at room temperature.

4. Urea standard solution (40 mg/dl)

Dissolve 1 gm (AR grade) dry urea in 50 ml of saturated solution of benzoic acid. Make up the volume to 100 ml with distilled water. Dilute 4 ml of the above stock solution up to 100 ml with saturated solution of benzoic acid. Store at 2–8° C.

Experiment 33

OBJECT

Quantitative determination of creatinine in blood/serum.

Reagents

Creatinine kit (J. Mitra and Co. Ltd.)
This kit contains the following reagents.
Creatinine reagent A (saturated picric acid solution).
Alkaline reagent.
Creatinine standard 150 mg/dl (stock solution).

Principle

Creatinine reacts with alkaline picrate to form red coloured complex. The optical density of red colour is proportional to the amount of creatinine in the sample which is measured at 520 ± 15 nm colorimetrically.

Creatinine + picric acid ⟶ orange coloured complex.

Procedure

Preparation of working standard solution: Dilute 0.1 ml of stock standard solution to 10 ml with distilled water.

Deproteinization of test sample

Sample/reagent	*Quantity*
Diluted urine/serum	1 ml
Distilled water	1 ml
Creatinine reagent A	6 ml

Mix well and put in boiling water bath for 1 minute. Cool and centrifuge for 5 minutes. Take three test tubes marked as B (blank), S (standard), and T (test).

S. no.	*Reagent*	*Blank*	*Standard*	*Test*
1.	Supernatant of the above	—	—	4 ml
2.	Working standard	—	1 ml	—
3.	Distilled water	1 ml	—	—
4.	Creatinine reagent A	3 ml	3 ml	—
5.	Alkali reagent	1 ml	1 ml	1 ml

Mix well and allow to stand at room temperature for 20 minutes. Measure the absorbance of blank, standard, and test against distilled water adjusted to zero at 520 nm.

Calculation

$$\text{Serum creatinine in mg/dl} = \frac{\text{OD of test sample} - \text{OD of blank}}{\text{OD of standard} - \text{OD of blank}} \times 3$$

Result

Normal value

Male	:	0.9–1.4 mg/dl
Female	:	0.8–1.2 mg/dl

Clinical significance

Increased level: Impaired renal functions.

Decreased level: Muscular dystrophy.

Reagents

1. *Alkaline picrate solution* (alkali reagent): To 10 ml of saturated solution, add 2 ml of 10% W/V of NaOH solution and mix. Store at room temperature.
2. *Creatinine standard solution* (150 mg/dl): Prepare the standard solution in 0.1 N HCl. Take pure creatinine and make the volume with 0.1 N HCl. Store at 2– 8° C.
3. *For deproteinization*: 10% W/V sodium tungstate solution and 2/3 N sulphuric acid are used in equal volume (creatinine reagent A). Store at room temperature.

Experiment 34

OBJECT

Quantitative determination of cholesterol in blood/serum.

Reagents

Cholesterol kit (J. Mitra Co. Ltd.) contains.

1. Cholesterol reagent (ferric perchlorate, ethyl acetate, and sulphuric acid solution).
2. Cholesterol standard (200 mg/dl): Dissolve 200 mg (AR grade) cholesterol in glacial acetic acid and make up the volume to 100 ml with glacial acetic acid. Store at room temperature.

Principle

Cholesterol reacts with hot solution of ferric ions, ethyl acetate and sulphuric acid (cholesterol reagent) to form purple coloured complex which is measured photometrically at 580 ± 15 nm.

Specimen

The sample should be collected from fasting individual. The use of heparin as anticoagulant is desirable.

Procedure

Take 3 dry and clean test tubes and marked as B (blank), S (standard), and T (test).

S. no.	*Reagents*	*Quantity*		
		B	*S*	*T*
1.	Cholesterol reagent	3 ml	3 ml	3 ml
2.	Distilled water	25 ml	—	—
3.	Cholesterol standard	—	25 μl	—
4.	Serum/plasma	—	—	25 μl

Add the reagents as above. Mix well. Put all the tubes in boiling water for exactly 90 seconds. Cool in cold water for 3 minutes. Adjust the instrument to zero with blank and take the optical densities of all tubes at 580 nm.

Calculation

$$\text{Total cholesterol in serum/plasma (mg/dl)} = \frac{\text{OD of test sample}}{\text{OD of standard}} \times 200$$

Result

Normal value: 150–250 mg/dl.

Diagnostic significance

High value may be found in athenosclerosis, diabetes mellitus, myxodema and obstructive jaundice, etc. Decreased levels are observed in hyperthyroidism, mal-absorption and anaemia.

Cholesterol reagent

In 2 litre RB flask, pour 520 mg ferric perchlorate (AR grade) and 600 ml of ethyl acetate. This flask is placed on a magnetic mixer containing teflon coated stirrer bar for stirring. Keep the temperature of the flask at 4° C by placing crushed ice around the flask. Continue the stirring until ferric per chlorate dissolves. From a separating funnel containing 400 ml of conc. H_2SO_4 (pre-chilled), add drop by drop conc. H_2SO_4 into the flask containing the ethyl acetate – ferric per chlorate solution. The temperature of the mixture does not exceed 45° C. It can be stored at room temperature.

Experiment 35

OBJECT

Quantitative determination of bilirubin in blood/serum.

Reagent

Bilirubin test kit (J. Mitra Co. Ltd.) contains the following reagents.

1. Diazo reagent A (sulphanilic acid solution).
2. Diazo reagent B (sodium nitrite solution).
3. Diazo blank (hydrochloric acid solution).
4. Bilirubin reagent D (methanol).
5. Bilirubin standard (10 mg/dl).

Principle

Bilirubin is found in two forms, conjugated and unconjugated forms. The conjugated bilirubin is called direct and unconjugated is called indirect. Estimation of bilirubin is based on its reaction with diazotized sulfanilic acid to form azobilirubin, a red purple coloured compound. In case of conjugated bilirubin it take place in acidic medium but in presence of methanol both bilirubins (conjugated and unconjugated) are diazotized. Thus, it gives the total bilirubin content in the sample. The intensity of purple colour that is formed is proportional to the bilirubin concentration in the serum.

Bilirubin + diazotized sulfanilic acid ⟶ Azobilirubin (red purple colour)

Specimen

Fresh serum should be used.

Procedure

Preparation of diazo working reagent (just before use): Mix 3.3 ml of diazo reagent A with 0.1 ml of diazo reagent B. Take 4 test tubes marked as T1 (total), T2 (total blank), D1 (direct), and D2 (direct blank).

S. no.	*Reagents*	*Quantity*			
		T1	*T2*	*D1*	*D2*
1.	Serum/plasma	0.2	0.2	0.2	0.2
2.	Distilled water	1.8	1.8	1.8	1.8
3.	Bilirubin diazo blank	—	0.5	—	0.5
4.	Diazo working reagent	0.5	—	0.5	—
5.	Distilled water	—	—	2.5	2.5
6.	Bilirubin reagent D	2.5	2.5	—	—

Mix well and read optical densities of D1 and D2 after 1 minute against distilled water adjusted to zero at 540 nm. Keep the tubes T1 and T2 in dark at room temperature for 30 minutes and measure the optical density of the both tubes (T1 and T2) against distilled water adjusted to zero at 540 nm.

Measurement of standard: Read the optical density of bilirubin standard against distilled water.

Calculation

$$\text{Total bilirubin in mg/dl} = \frac{\text{OD of T1} - \text{OD of T2}}{\text{OD of standard}} \times 10$$

$$\text{Direct bilirubin in mg/dl} = \frac{\text{OD of D1} - \text{OD of D2}}{\text{OD of standard}} \times 10$$

Indirect = Total – direct bilirubin

Normal value
Adults (total) : 0.2 – 1 mg/dl
(direct) : 0 – 0.2 mg/dl

Result

Diagnostic significance

Increase levels: Liver diseases, Coombs position anaemia, defective uptake and storage of bilirubin, defective glucuronyl transferase activity.

Reagents

1. *Diazo reagent A* (sulphanilic acid solution): Add 5 gm of sulphanilic acid to 60 ml of conc. HCl in a litre of VF and dilute to the mark with distilled water. Store at room temperature.
2. *Diazo reagent B* (sodium nitrite solution): Dissolve 20 gm sodium nitrite ($NaNO_2$) in distilled water and dilute to the volume of 100 ml with distilled water. Store at 2 to 8° C.
3. *Bilirubin standard* (10 mg/dl): Dissolve 100 mg in 100 ml of distilled water. Dilute 10 ml of the stock solution to 100 ml with distilled water. Store at 2 to 8° C.
4. *Diazo blank*: Dilute 60 ml of conc. HCl to 1 litre with distilled water. Store at room temperature.
5. *Bilirubin reagent D* (methanol): Analytical grade. Store at room temperature.

Experiment 36

OBJECT

Quantitative determination of calcium in blood/serum by titrimetric method.

Reagents

1. *Sodium edetate stock solution* (0.05 M): Weigh 14.8 gm of disodium EDTA dihydrate in to 1 litre volumetric flask. Add distilled water to dissolve and finally make the volume up to 1 litre with distilled water.
2. NaOH (2N).
3. *Indicator*: Eriochrome or methyl-thymol blue.
4. *Calcium standard* (0.4 mg/ml): Weigh 0.1 gm of anhydrous calcium carbonate (previously dried 110° C and cool in a dessicator) in volumetric flask containing 20 ml of distilled water and 2 ml of 1 NHCl. Heat to dissolve the content and cool. Dilute to 100 ml with distilled water.

Specimen

Serum or heparinized plasma should be collected in fasting state.

Principle

The calcium of the specimen is titrated against sodium EDTA which forms complex and removes calcium from the titrating fluid which change the colour of the indicator. The EDTA is standardized by titrating with standard calcium.

$$\text{Calcium conc. in serum in mg/dl} = \frac{\text{Volume of titrant (EDTA) needed for the test solution}}{\text{Volume of the titrant (EDTA) needed for the standard solution}} \times 10$$

m mol/litre = mg/dl × 0.25

Procedure

Working EDTA solution: Take 2 ml of stock solution and is diluted to 100 ml with distilled water.

Working standard solution of calcium (10 mg/dl): Dilute 25 ml of stock solution to 100 ml with distilled water. Take two clean and dry conical flasks and marked as T and S. Add 1 ml of serum in the flask mark T and 1 ml of working standard solution of calcium (0.1 mg) in the S marked flask. Add 4 ml of NaOH and 25 ml of distilled water to each flask. Put 2 drops of indicator in each flask. Fill the burette with diluted sodium edetate solution and titrate the contents of the flask until colour changes from purple to light blue. The volume of titrant is noted for test and standard solution.

Result

Normal value: 9–12 mg/dl (2.2 to 3 milli mole/litre).

Clinical significance

Increase levels: It is observed in parathyroid diseases, vitamin D in-balance, multiple myeloma and neoplastic diseases.

Low levels: It is found in osteomalacia, rickets and renal failure, etc.

6

Enzymology

Enzymes are powerful biocatalysts. All enzymes are protein in nature. Most of the enzymes are conjugated proteins, i.e. protein is associated with some non-protein component called a cofactor. The protein part of the enzyme is called apoenzyme. The cofactor may be metal ions like Zn^{2+}, Mg^{2+}, Fe^{2+}, Cu^{2+}, etc. and organic non-protein molecules (coenzyme). The activity of enzymes are maximum at optimum pH and temperature. At international level the enzymes are classified on basis of types of reactions which they catalyze.

1. Transferases

They catalyze the transfer of various groups from one molecule to another, e.g. transaminases and transphosphorylases, etc.

Transaminases

They bring about transamination which is a process in which an amino group is transferred from one amino acid to an α-ketoacid. The diagnostically useful transaminases are glutamate oxaloacetate transaminase (GOT) and glutamate pyruvate transaminase (GPT).

Clinical significance

Increases serum transaminase activity is seen in liver dysfunction. The greater activity GOT over GPT is typical of myocardial infaraction.

Normal range

SGOT : 5 – 40 u/l.
SGPT : 5 – 35 u/l.

2. Hydrolases

They catalyze the hydrolases of substrates, e.g. phosphates, lipases, proteinases, and carbohydrases, etc.

Phosphates

They hydrolyze a large variety of organic phosphate esters with the formation of an alcohol and phosphate ions, e.g. alkaline phosphatase and acid phosphatase.

The pH of measuring the alkaline phosphatase activity is 10 and for acid phosphatase it is 5.

Acid phosphatase

It is found in RBC, WBC, prostate, and platelets, etc. In small amount it is found in liver bone and kidney also. Its level is increased in cancer of prostate.

Normal range

1–4 KA units/dl.

Alkaline phosphatase

It is found in liver, bone, placenta, and intestine. The highest level is found in hyperparathyroidism. It's level rises moderately in osteomalacia. The enzyme level is considerably increased in inflammatory diseases and metastatic carcinoma of liver, biliary cirrhosis, and hepatitis.

Normal range

Adult : 4–17 KA/dl.
Children : 15–33 KA/dl.

Amylases

It is an amylolytic enzyme, hydrolyzes the starch and amylose to maltose. The salivary gland and pancreas produce amylase may release into circulation in certain pathological condition. Its serum level is raised in peptic ulcer, empyema of gall bladder, intestinal obstruction, peritonitis, etc. The urinary amylase is raised in a acute pancreatitis. It can be estimated by either measuring the amount of maltose released per unit time or by measuring the disappearance of the starch.

Lipase

It catalyzes the hydrolysis of esters to form fatty acid and monoglycerides.

Clinical Significance

It is secreted by pancreas and may appear in the circulation in acute pancreatitis. It is also raised in biliary disease, peptic ulcer and caner of pancreas.

Normal range

Up to 1.5 units/ml in serum.

Estimation by titration method

Quantitavely lipase activity can be determined by measuring the fatty acids released by the serum lipase from an olive oil as substrate. These are titrated with sodium hydroxide using thymol-phthalein as the indicator.

Reagents

Olive oil emulsion, NaOH (0.05 N), thymol-phthalein, ethyl alcohol 95% and barbiturate buffer pH 8.

Procedure

Take two flask marked as T (test) and B (blank). At 3 ml of olive oil emulsion, 1 ml buffer solution and 3 ml distilled water in both the flasks and incubate them in a water bath at 37° C for 6 hours. Add 3 ml 95% alcohol and 2 drops of indicators into both the flasks. Titrate the both contents of the flasks with 0.05 N NaOH taking in burette. At the end point the colour is blue. Subtract the blank reading from the test value.

Units of lipase = VT – VB × 0.05.
VT = Volume of NaOH in ml consumed for test flask.
VB = Volume of NaOH in ml consumed for blank.

3. Oxidases and reductases (dehydrogenases)

They catalyze redox, reactions, e.g. LDH (lactate dehydrogenase).

4. Lyases

They catalyze bound cleavage.

5. Isomerases

They catalyze isomerisation reactions.

6. Ligases

They catalyze the formation of single bond in presence of ATP.

Experiment 37

OBJECT

Quantitative determination of alkaline phosphatase in serum or plasma.

Alkaline phosphatase kit (J. Mitra Co. Ltd.) contains the following reagents.

Reagent A: Buffer substrate (pH 10).

Reagent B: Sodium hydroxide.

Reagent C: Sodium bicarbonate.

Reagent D: 4-amino-antipyrine.

Reagent E: Potassium ferricyanide.

Phenol standard (stock 1 mg/ml).

All of the above reagents can be stored at 2– 8° C for stability of 1 year.

Specimen collection

Serum or plasma (heparinized) can be used. Anticoagulant like oxalate, citrate and EDTA inhibit the enzyme activity, hence not recommended. The serum sample should be collected from a fasting individual.

Unit

The activity of enzyme is expressed in king Armstrong (KA).

Principle

Phosphatases bring about hydrolysis of organic phosphate compounds. Phosphatase are of two kinds, i.e. alkaline phosphatase and acid phosphatase. There activity is differentiated in alkaline and acidic medium at pH 10 and 5 respectively.

For estimation of alkaline phosphatase serum is incubated with phenyl phosphate buffered at pH 10 for 15 minutes at 37° C. The hydrolysis product phenol is condensed with 4-amino-antipyrin which is then oxidized with alkaline ferricyanide to give red coloured complex which is measured colorimetrically at 520 nm.

$$\text{Phenyl phosphate} \xrightarrow[\text{pH 10}]{\text{Alkaline phosphatase}} \text{Phenol + Pi}$$

$$\text{Phenol + 4-amino-antipyrin} \xrightarrow[\text{OH}^-]{\text{Potassium ferricyanide}} \text{Orange red coloured complex}$$

Procedure

Preparation of working buffer solution – Reconstitute 1 vial of buffer substrate with 9 ml distilled water and mix it well (stable for 15 days).

Preparation of working phenol standard (0.01 mg/ml) – Dilute 0.1 ml of stock solution to 10 ml with distilled water (stable for 8 – 10 hours at room temperature).

Take four test tubes and proceed as follow:

S.no.	Reagent	Quantity in ml			
		B	S	C	T
1.	Reagent A	—	—	2 ml	2 ml
2.	Distilled water	2 ml	1.1 ml	—	—
			Incubate at 37° C for 15 minutes		
3.	Working standard solution	—	1 ml	—	—
4.	Serum	—	—	—	0.05 ml
			Incubate at 37° C for 15 minutes		
5.	Reagent B	0.4 ml	0.4 ml	0.4 ml	0.4 ml
6.	Serum	—	—	0.05 ml	—
7.	Reagent C	0.5 ml	0.5 ml	0.5 ml	0.5 ml
8.	Reagent D	0.5 ml	0.5 ml	0.5 ml	0.5 ml
9.	Reagent E	0.5 ml	0.5 ml	0.5 ml	0.5 ml

Mix well. Keep them for 20 minutes at room temperature. Measure absorbance of all tubes at 520 nm against distilled water adjusted to zero.

Calculation

$$\text{Alkaline phosphatase (KA units/dl)} = \frac{\text{OD of test} - \text{OD of control}}{\text{OD of standard} - \text{OD of blank}} \times 20$$

Where OD = optical density (absorbance).
In S tube 1 ml of working standard solution = 0.01 mg of phenol.
Here serum taken 0.05 ml librates 0.01 mg of phenol.

So $$100 \text{ ml of serum} = \frac{0.01}{0.05} \times 100 = 20 \text{ mg of phenol}$$

So $$\frac{\text{OD of test} - \text{OD of control}}{\text{OD of standard} - \text{OD of blank}} \text{ is multiplied by } 20$$

1 KA unit is the formation of 1 mg of phenol in 15 minutes under the condition of the test.

Normal range

Adults : 4–17 KA units/dl.
Children : 17–33 KA units/dl.

Result

Diagnostic significance

Increased levels are found in hepato-biliary, bone diseases, Hodgkin's disease. CCF and infective hepatitis.

Decreased levels are seen in anaemia, scurvy, kwashiorkor and cretinism.

Experiment 38

OBJECT

Quantitative determination of acid phosphatase in serum or plasma.

Acid phosphatase kit (J. Mitra Co. Ltd.) contains the following reagents.

Reagent A: Buffer substrate (pH 5).

Reagent B: Sodium hydroxide.

Reagent C: Sodium bicarbonate.

Reagent D: 4-amino-antipyrine.

Reagent E: Potassium ferricyanide.

Phenol standard (stock 1 mg/ml).

All the above reagents can be stored at 2– 8° C for stability of 1 year.

Specimen collection

Serum or plasma (heparinized) can be used. Anticoagulant like oxalate, citrate and EDTA inhibit the enzyme activity, hence not recommended. The serum sample should be collected from a fasting individual.

Unit

The activity of enzyme is expressed in king Armstrong (KA).

Principle

Acid phosphatase brings about hydrolysis of phenyl phosphate at pH 5 for 60 minutes at 37° C. The hydrolysed product phenol is reacted with 4-amino-antipyrine in presence of potassium ferricyanide to form orange red colour complex which is estimated colorimetrically at 520 nm.

$$\text{Phenyl phosphate} \xrightarrow[\text{pH 5}]{\text{Alkaline phosphatase}} \text{Phenol + Pi}$$

$$\text{Phenol + 4-amino-antipyrin} \xrightarrow[\text{OH}^-]{\text{Potassium ferricyanide}} \text{Orange red coloured complex}$$

Procedure

Preparation of working buffer solution: Reconstitute 1 vial of buffer substrate with 9 ml distilled water and mix it well (stable for 7 days).

Preparation of working phenol standard (0.01 mg/ml): Dilute 0.1 ml of stock solution to 10 ml with distilled water (stable for 8–10 hours at room temperature).

Take four test tubes and proceed as follow:

S.no.	Reagent	Quantity in ml			
		B	S	C	T
1.	Reagent A	—	—	2 ml	2 ml
2.	Distilled water	2 ml	1.1 ml	—	—
			Incubate at 37° C for 3 minutes		
3.	Working standard solution	—	1 ml	—	—
4.	Serum	—	—	—	0.1 ml
			Incubate at 37° C for 60 minutes		
5.	Reagent B	0.5 ml	0.5 ml	0.5 ml	0.5 ml
6.	Serum	—	—	0.1 ml	—
7.	Reagent C	0.5 ml	0.5 ml	0.5 ml	0.5 ml
8.	Reagent D	0.5 ml	0.5 ml	0.5 ml	0.5 ml
9.	Reagent E	0.5 ml	0.5 ml	0.5 ml	0.5 ml

Mix well. Keep them for 5 minutes at room temperature. Measure absorbance of all tubes at 520 nm against distilled water adjusted to zero.

Calculation

$$\text{Acid phosphatase (KA units/dl)} = \frac{\text{OD of test} - \text{OD of control}}{\text{OD of standard}} \times 10$$

Where OD = optical density (absorbance).
In S tube 1 ml of working standard solution = 0.01 mg of phenol.
Here serum taken 0.1 ml librates 0.01 mg of phenol.

So $$\text{100 ml of serum} = \frac{0.01}{0.1} \times 100 = \text{10 mg of phenol}$$

So $$\frac{\text{OD of test} - \text{OD of control}}{\text{OD of standard}} \text{ is multiplied by } 10$$

Normal range

1–4 KA units/dl.

Result

Diagnostic significance

Increased levels are found in cancer of prostate, Gaucher's diseses, hyper parathyroidism, multiple myeloma, hepatitis, obstructive jaundice, haemolytic anaemia and Paget's disease.

Reagents

For alkaline phosphatase

1. ***Buffer substrate solution* pH 10:** Mix equal volume of solution A and B.

Solution A: Disodium phenyl phosphate (0.001M) Dissolve 2.18 gm in 1 litre of distilled water. Boil the solution and cool. Add chloroform (4 ml/litre) to preserve it. Store at 4° C.

Solution B: (Buffer pH 10)—6.3 gm of anhydrous sodium carbonate 3.36 gm of sodium bicarbonate in 1 litre distilled water. Store at 4° C.

2. NaOH (0.5N).
3. $NaHCO_3$ (0.5 N).
4. Potassium ferrocyanide (2.4% W/V): Store in brown bottle.
5. 4-amino-antipyrine solution (0.6% W/V): Store in brown bottle.
6. Standard phenol stock solution (1 mg/ml): Dissolve 100 mg of AR grade phenol in 100 ml of 0.1 NaOH.

For acid phosphatase

Citrate buffer pH 5: Dissolve 42 gm of crystalline citric acid in distilled water, add 376 ml of N NaOH and make up the volume of 1 litre with distilled water. Store at 4° C. To prepare buffer substrate solution mix equal volume of citrate buffer pH 5 and disodium phenol phosphate (0.001 M).

Experiment 39

OBJECT

Quantitative determination of SGOT (serum glutamic oxaloacetate transaminase).

Reagents

This kit (ACE Diagnostics and Biotech Ltd.) contains the following reagents.

Reagent 1: Substrate reagent (L aspartic acid) – 33 mM/litre and 2-oxoglutarate – 05 mM/litre.

Reagent 2: SGOT colour reagent (2, 4-dianitrophenyl hydrazyne) 1 mM/litre.

Reagent 3: Calibrator (sodium pyruvate) – 150 U/litre.

Reagent 4: Alkali reagent (sodium hydroxide)— 4 N.

Specimen

Unhemolyzed serum.

Principle

SGOT is transaminase enzyme which brings about transamination. SGOT catalyzes the transfer of amino group from aspartic acid to oxoglutarate to form oxaloacetate and L-glutamate. The oxaloacetate thus formed reacts with 2, 4-dinitrophenyle hydrazine to form a corresponding hydrazone, a brownish red colour complex in an alkaline medium. It is measured colorimetrically at 520 nm or with green filter.

L-aspartate + α-keto-glutarate $\longrightarrow$ oxaloacetate + L-glutamate

Commercially, available kit of J. Mitra Co. Ltd. for quantitative determination of SGOT involves the preparation of standard calibration curve (graph) from which SGOT unit of sample is calculated. Other kit of ACE Diagnostics and Biotech Ltd. mentions the procedure without graph.

Procedure

Working alkali reagent: Dilute the alkali reagent 1 ml with 9 ml distilled water. Pipette in four test tubes marked as B (blank), CL (calibrator), C (control), and T (test).

S.no.	Reagent	Quantity in ml			
		B	CL	C	T
1.	Substrate reagent	0.5	0.5	0.5	0.5
2.	Distilled water	0.1	—	—	—
3.	Sample	—	—	—	0.1
4.	Calibrator	—	0.1 ml	—	—
		Mix and incubate at 37° C for 60 minutes			
5.	SGOT colour reagent	0.5	0.5	0.5	0.5
6.	Sample	—	—	0.1 ml	—
		Mix and incubate for 20 minutes at room temperature			
7.	Alkali reagent (diluted)	3 ml	3 ml	3 ml	3 ml

Read the optical density of all test tubes against distilled water at 520 nm or with green filter.

Calculation

$$\text{SGOT (AST) activity in U/L} = \frac{\text{OD of test} - \text{OD of control}}{\text{OD of calibrator} - \text{OD of blank}} \times \text{conc. of calibrator}$$

Normal range

5 – 40 U/litre.

Clinical significance

Increased levels are observed myocardial infarction, liver cel! damage and muscular dystrophy.

Experiment 40

OBJECT

Quantitative determination of SGPT (serum glutamic pyruvic transaminase).

Reagents

This kit (ACE Diagnostics and Biotech Ltd.) contains the following reagents.

Reagent 1: Substrate reagent (L-alanine)–200 mM/litre and 2 oxoglutarate–02 mM/litre.
Reagent 2: SGPT colour reagent (2,4-dianitrophenyl hydrazyne) 1 mM/litre.
Reagent 3: Calibrator (sodium pyruvate)–170 U/litre.
Reagent 4: Alkali reagent (sodium hydroxide)—4 N.

Specimen

Unhemolyzed serum.

Principle

SGPT is transaminase enzyme which brings about transamination. It catalyzes the transfer of the amino group from L-alanine to α-keto-glutarate to form pyruvate and L-glutamate. The pyruvate thus formed reacts with 2, 4-dinitrophenyl hydrazine to form a corresponding hydrazone, a brownish red colour complex in an alkaline medium. It is measured colorimetrically at 520 nm or with green filter.

L-alanine + α-keto-glutarate ⟶ pyruvate + L-glutamate

Commercially, available kit of J. Mitra Co. Ltd. for quantitative determination of SGPT involves the preparation of standard calibration curve (graph) from which SGPT unit of sample is calculated. Other kit of ACE Diagnostics and Biotech Ltd. mentions the procedure without graph.

Procedure

Working alkali reagent: Dilute the alkali reagent 1 ml with 9 ml distilled water. Pipette in four test tubes marked as B (blank), CL (calibrator), C (control), and T (test).

S.no.	*Reagent*	*Quantity in ml*			
		B	*CL*	*C*	*T*
1.	Substrate reagent	0.5	0.5	0.5	0.5
2.	Distilled water	0.1	—	—	—
3.	Sample (serum)	—	—	—	0.1
4.	Calibrator	—	0.1 ml	—	—
		Mix and incubate at 37° C for 30 minutes			
5.	SGPT colour reagent	0.5	0.5	0.5	0.5
6.	Sample (serum)	—	—	0.1 ml	—
		Mix and incubate for 20 minutes at room temperature			
7.	Alkali reagent (diluted)	3 ml	3 ml	3 ml	3 ml

Read the optical density of all test tubes against distilled water at 520 nm or with green filter.

Calculation

$$\text{SGPT (ALT) activity in U/L} = \frac{\text{OD of test} - \text{OD of control}}{\text{OD of calibrator} - \text{OD of blank}} \times \text{conc. of calibrator}$$

Where OD is optical density.

Normal range

5–35 U/litre.

Clinical significance

Increased levels are observed in liver diseases, i.e. obstructive jaundice, carcinoma of liver and hepatitis.

Experiment 41

OBJECT

Quantitative determination of SGPT/SGOT by calibration curve method.

Reagents

SGOT/SGPT (J. Mitra Co. Ltd.) kit contains the following reagents.

1. *Solution A*: SGOT buffer substrate powder reconstitute each vial with 5 ml of distilled water.
2. *Solution A*: SGPT buffer substrate powder reconstitute each vial with 5 ml of distilled water.
3. *Solution B*: DNPH colour developer.
4. *Solution C*: Conc. sodium hydroxide solution (0.4 N).
5. SGOT calibration standard solution (2 mmol/litre).
6. SGPT calibration standard solution (2 mmol/litre).

Principle

SGOT is transaminase enzyme which brings about transamination. SGOT catalyzes the transfer of amino group from aspartic acid to oxoglutarate to form oxaloacetate and L-glutamate. The oxaloacetate thus formed reacts with 2, 4-dinitrophenyl hydrazine to form a corresponding hydrazone, a brownish red colour complex in an alkaline medium. It is measured colorimetrically at 520 nm or with green filter.

L-aspartate + α-keto-glutarate ⟶ oxaloacetate + L-glutamate

SGPT is transaminase enzyme which brings about transamination. It catalyzes the transfer of the amino group from L-alanine to α-keto-glutarate to form pyruvate and L-glutamate. The pyruvate thus formed reacts with 2, 4-dinitrophenyl hydrazine to form a corresponding hydrazone, a brownish red colour complex in an alkaline medium. It is measured colorimetrically at 520 nm or with green filter.

L-alanine + α-keto-glutarate ⟶ pyruvate + L-glutamate

Procedure

Preparation of calibration curve: Take working substrate buffer (SGOT/SGPT), pyruvate working standard (2 m mol/litre) and distilled water as shown in table below.

Tube no.	*Working substrate buffer (ml)*	*Working standard (2 m mol/litre)*	*Distilled water*	*SGOT units*	*SGPT units*
1.	0.05	0.00	0.1	0	0
2.	0.45	0.05	0.1	24	28
3.	0.40	0.10	0.1	61	57
4.	0.35	0.15	0.1	114	97
5.	0.3	0.2	0.1	190	157

To each tube, add 0.5 ml of DNPH. Mix and allow to stand for 20 minutes. After 20 minutes add 5 ml of 0.4 N NaOH solution to all test tubes and keep for 10 minutes at room temperature. Take the optical density of all the test tubes at 520 nm against distilled water adjusted to zero. To prepare the curve plot OD against SGOT/SGPT units.

For test solution

Reagents	Quantity
Working buffer solution	0.5 ml (incubate at 37° C for 5 minutes)
Serum	0.1 (for SGOT incubate at 37° C for 60 minutes and for SGPT incubate at 37° C for 30 minutes)
DNPH	0.5 (mix well and allow to stand at room temperature for 20 minutes)
NaOH solution (0.4 N)	5 ml (mix well and allow to stand at room temperature for 10 minutes)

Note: The optical densities of the solution at 520 nm against distilled water adjusted to zero.

Calculation

From OD of test, calculate the SGOT/SGPT unit from standard curve. If units exceed from 100 the serum can be diluted to 4 times and multiply the result by 4 to get final result.

Normal range

SGOT : 10–40 units
SGPT : 1–53 units

Result

Reagents

1. *Phosphate buffer 7.4, 0.1 M:* 7.5 gm of dry anhydrous disodium hydrogen phosphate and 1.81 gm of dry anhydrous potassium dihydrogen phosphate per litre in distilled water. Check the pH and store at 4° C. Disodium hydrogen phosphate increases the pH, while potassium dihydrogen phosphate decrease the pH.
2. *Substrate for SGOT DL aspartate (200 mmol/litre) and α-keto-glutarate (2 mmol/litre)*: Dissolve 2.66 gm aspartic acid and 30 mg of oxoglutaric acid in 20.5 ml of 1 N NaOH place in 250 ml of beaker. Adjust the pH to 7.4 by adding NaOH 0.1 N drop by drop. Transfer the contents in volumetric flask (100 ml). Make up the volume to 100 ml with phosphate buffer solution 7.4 pH. Store at 2– 4° C, add 1 ml chloroform as preservative.
3. *Substrate SGPT*: 1.78 gm of DL-alanine and 30 mg of oxoglutaric acid in 20 ml of phosphate buffer containing 1.25 ml of 0.4 N NaOH. Make up the volume up to 100 ml with phosphate buffer and adjust the pH to 7.4. Add 1 ml of chloroform as preservative. Store at 2– 4° C.

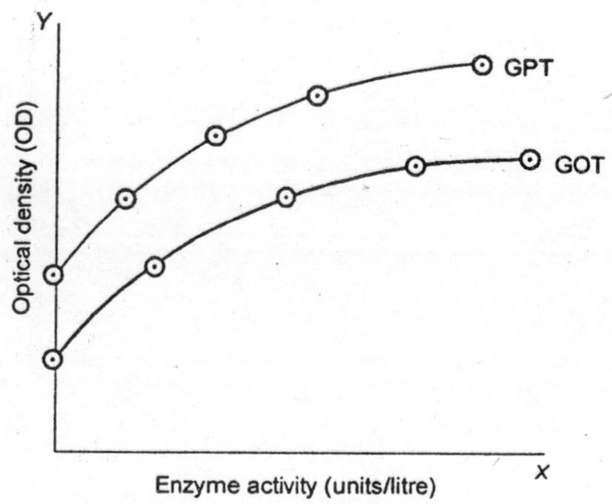

4. *Pyruvate standard (Stock solution 20 mmol/litre)*: Dissolve 220 mg sodium pyruvate in phosphate buffer solution and make up the volume up to 100 ml.

   Working pyruvate standard (2 mmol/litre): Dilute 10 ml of stock solution to 100 ml with phosphate buffer.
5. *2, 4-dinitrophenyl hydrazine (DNPH) 1 mmol/litre*: Dissolve 200 mg DNPH in 1 N HCl (heat if necessary) and make up to 1 litre with 1 N HCl. Store at 2– 4° C.
6. *NaOH.* 0 4 N, 1 N

   1 N NaOH: Dissolve 40 gm in distilled water and make up the volume to 1 litre with distilled water.

   0.4 N NaOH: Dilute 40 ml of 1 N NaOH to 100 ml with distilled water.

7

Examination of Sputum

Sputum is the tracheobronchial exudate or excretory product which consists of plasma, water, electrolytes, and mucus.

Collection: The specimen should be collected in sterile container. Generally, the first morning sputum is preferred. The mouth should be rinsed firstly before collecting the sputum to avoid contaminants from oral cavity.

Physical Examination

1. Quantity

Large quantity is found in tuberculosis, lung abscess, bronchietasis and chronic bronchitis whereas less quantity is evident in acute bronchitis.

2. Colour

Normal sputum	:	Colourless
Yellow colour	:	Indicates pus and epithelial cells.
Green	:	Pseudomonas infection and jaundice.
Black	:	Due to inhalation of dust and coal dust.
Red	:	Due to fresh blood as in haemorrhage and mitral stenosis.
Brown	:	Pulmonary gangrene, pneumonia.

3. Appearance

a. *Serous*: Colourless or yellow as in pulmonary edema.
b. *Purulent pus*: As in bronchiectasis.
c. *Bloody*: As in mitral stenosis, lung cancer, tuberculosis.
d. *Mucoid*: As in asthma, pneumonia and whooping cough.

4. Odour

a. *Normal sputum*: Odourless.
b. *Putrid odour*: Lung abscess, gangrene and tuberculosis.

Microscopic examination

Non-stained sputum

1. Curschmann's spirals
2. Elastic fibres
3. Crystals, i.e. charcot leyden, fatty acid, cholesterol, leucin and tyrosine.
4. Casts
5. Pigments
6. Myelin globules
7. Malignant cells
8. Parasites

Stained sputum for bacteriological examination

- AFB (acid fast bacteria), i.e. mycobacterium tuberculosis (by Ziehl Nelson Method)
- Gram staining, i.e. streptococci, staphylococci, diplococci, diphtheria

1. **Curschmann's spiral:** It is made up of twisted strands of mucus enclosing leucocytes, e.g. bronchial asthma.
2. **Elastic fibres:** Their presence indicates the lung abscess and damage of parenchymatous cells of lung.
3. **Crystals**
   a. *Charcot leyden crystals*: It is colourless or yellowish, octahedral crystals which stain with eosin, e.g. bronchial asthma.
   b. *Fatty acid crystals*: It is found in gangrene and chronic tuberculosis.
   c. *Cholesterol crystals:* It is found in chronic lung abscess and chronic tuberculosis.
   d. *Leucin and tyrosin crystals*: These are the break down product of proteins. They indicate the damage of lung.
4. **Casts:** These are found in fibrinous bronchitis.
5. **Pigments:** These are found in pulmonary infarction.
6. **Myelin globules:** These are seen in mucoid sputum. They result from degeneration of alveolar epithelium, e.g. bronchitis.
7. **Malignant cells:** These are seen in pulmonary neoplasm.
8. **Parasites:** E.g. hydatid cyst, *E. histolytica*, etc.

Gram Staining

A smear of the sputum is prepared on the slides and is fixed by heating over a flame.

Smear → Treat with crystal violet (for 3 minutes) → Gram iodine (for 1 minutes) → Wash and treat with ethanol → Wash again in running water → Apply saffranin (for ½ minute) → Wash and dry → Examine it under oil immersion lens

Ziehl Nelson Method

For detection of AFB (acid fast bacteria), i.e. mycobacterium tuberculosis

The cell wall of this bacteria is made of mycolic acid, i.e. a high molecular weight hydroxy acid containing carboxyl groups. Hot strong carbol fuchsin is able to penetrate the bacterial cell wall and thus stains the bacteria. 20% H_2SO_4 cannot decolourize the acid fast bacilli while other organism and background substances are decolourized and stained blue with methylene blue.

Procedure

A smear of sputum is prepared on the slide and is fixed by heating over flame.

Smear	Pour hot strong carbol-fuchsin on smear or gently heat from below → wait for 5 minutes	Wash the slide and treat with 20% H_2SO_4 → for 1 minute	Again wash with water and counter stain with methylene blue → for 1 minute	Wash with water and dry →	Examine it under oil immersion lens without cover slip

Observation

Mycobacterium bacilli are seen as purple red rods. Other organisms and background stain blue.

Experiment 42

OBJECT

To carry out physical and microscopic examination of sputum.

Name of the patient/individual : ____________ Date : ____________
Age : ____________ Sex : ____________
Referred by : ____________

Physical examination

Colour : ____________
Apperance : ____________
Odour : ____________

Microscopic examination (unstained)

Curschmann's spirals : ____________
Elastic fibre : ____________
Crystals : ____________
Casts : ____________
Pigments : ____________
Myelin globules : ____________
Malignant cells : ____________
Parasites : ____________

Microscopic examination (stained)

AFB : ____________
Gram staining : ____________

Result

Interpretation

8

Examination of Faeces (Stool)

The stool is undigested materials of diet which is semisolid in consistency. It may contain traces of digested food also. Examination of stool has got many clinical and diagnostic values. The amount of adult stool is nearly 150–250 gm/day.

Collection: A freshly passed stool free from urine should be collected in wide mouth container or jar with a cap.

Interfering factors: Meat, barium, bismuth, oil and antibiotics.

Examination of faeces consists of:

1. Macroscopic examination.
2. Microscopic examination.

Macroscopic Examination

a. Colour

Normal : Brown.

Green: Intake of spinach, calomel or biliverdin.

Clay: Obstructive jaundice, pancreatic diseases and barium sulphate.

Black: Iron, bismuth, charcoal, blood.

b. Odour with reaction

Normal : Characteristic and reaction is neutral to slight alkaline.

Foul smell : Acute enteritis, alkaline reaction is due to putrefaction of protein.

Rancid odour : Acidic reaction due to carbohydrate fermentation.

c. Pus

Normal : Absent.

Abnormal : Presence of pus is indicative of chronic bacillary dysentery and ulcerative colitis.

d. Blood

Normal: Absent.

Abnormal: The presence of blood in stool is seen in the following diseases, i.e. peptic ulcer, gastritis, esophagitis, ulcerative colitis, carcinoma, heamorrhoids and fissure, etc.

e. Mucus

Normal: Absent or slight in amount.

Abnormal: Bloody mucus is found in neoplasm and inflammation of rectal canal while mucus with pus and blood is seen in ulcerative colitis, bacillary dysentery and carcinoma of colon.

f. Parasites

In normal stool parasites are absent. In worm infection, i.e. tapeworm segment, ascaris, pinworm, etc. are visible.

Microscopic Examination

Take a small amount of stool on a slide and is mixed with saline solution. Cover with cover slip and examine under microscope (10*x* × 40*x* objectives). It can be stained with iodine solution (for identification of starch cells and amoebic cysts) or with Sudan (for fat droplets).

a. *Erythrocytes*: Its presence indicates bleeding in intestine.
b. *Leucocytes*: These are seen in intestinal infection.
c. Epithelial cells, pus cells, macrophages also should be reported.
d. *Crystals*: Calcium oxalate, fatty acid, charcot lelyden crystal (needle shaped crystals seen in ulcerative condition of dysentery), haematoidin crystals (brownish needle as in case of heamorrhage).
e. *Parasites*: The microscopic examination for helminthics in stool has got great clinical significance. The helminthic eggs can be seen in stool of man. But concentration technique is preferred for final diagnosis.

Formol Saline Sedimentation Method

Formaldehyde saline solution (90 ml saline solution + 10 ml 40% w/v formaldehyde solution)–Mix the small quantity of stool in 10 ml of formaldehyde saline solution in a test tube. Pass it through sieve in to a beaker. Take 6 ml of suspension in to a centrifuge tube and add 3 ml of ether. Centrifuge at 3000 rpm/minute for one minute. The bottom of centrifuge tube contains deposit of parasites. Remove all the upper three layers (ether at top, stool particles at middle, formol saline in lower). Transfer the deposit on the slide and cover with cover slip. Examine under microscope (10*x* × 40*x* objectives). Different helmenthic eggs can be identify by their morphological characters as shown in figure below.

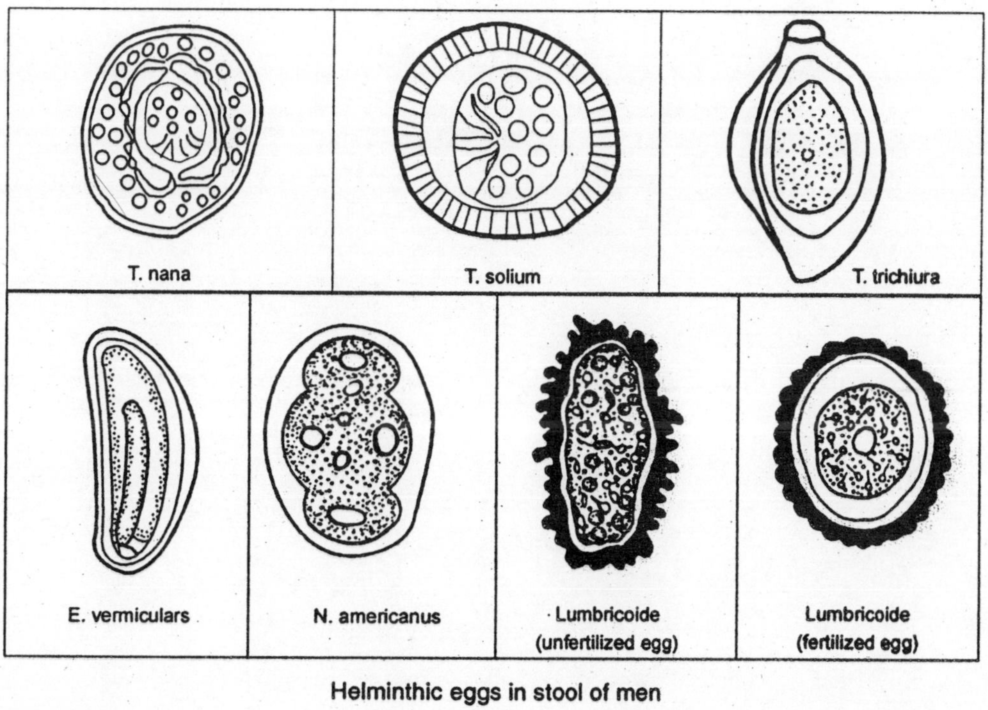

Helminthic eggs in stool of men

Experiment 43

OBJECT

Examination of faeces (macroscopic and microscopic) of human.

Date : ________________
Patient's name : ________________
Age : ________________
Sex : ________________
Referred by : ________________

Macroscopic Examination

Colour : ________________
Odour : ________________
Pus : ________________
Blood : ________________
Mucous : ________________
Parasites : ________________

Microscopic Examination

Erythrocytes : ________________
Leucocytes : ________________
Pus cells : ________________
Epithelial cells : ________________
Macrophages : ________________
Crystals : ________________
Parasites : (a) Direct specimen of stool

(b) Deposit of parasites by sedimentation technique

Result

Clinical significance

9

Injection of Drugs and Withdrawal of Blood Samples

Practice of injecting drugs can be learnt by student pharmacists during their practical training under the supervision of doctors, nurses or apprentice masters. The practical training (not less than 500 hours spread over a period of not less than 3 months) is a part of their curriculum as stated in ER-91.

Drug administration (parenteral): The parenteral (par-beyond; enterone-intestine) route of drug administration is rapid, reliable and emergency route, although this route needs special equipment and techniques. In all the circumstances where oral medications are failed, this route is preferred. There are three common routes which are widely employed.

1. *Subcutaneous*: Here needle (25–28 gauge) is used for administering 0.5 to 2 ml of drugs. The site of injection is usually outer surface of upper arm but sometimes anterior surface of thigh, abdomen or buttock can be used. Moist the skin with cotton treated with 70% alcohol and pinch between forefinger and thumb. The needle is inserted at a 45° angle to the skin, e.g. insulin injection.

2. *Intramuscular* (IM): In this route the drug is injected slowly in deltoid muscles, gluteal or thigh muscles. After inserting the needle, the plunger is drawn back gently to check vein puncture (blood is sucked back in the syringe). If it happens withdraw the needle. Aseptic technique must be followed.

3. *Intravenous* (IV): The vein (median cubital, basilic anterior, cephalic anterior and ulnar vein of forearm) is punctured slowly and steadily under asceptic precautions by sterile needle of gauge less than 22.

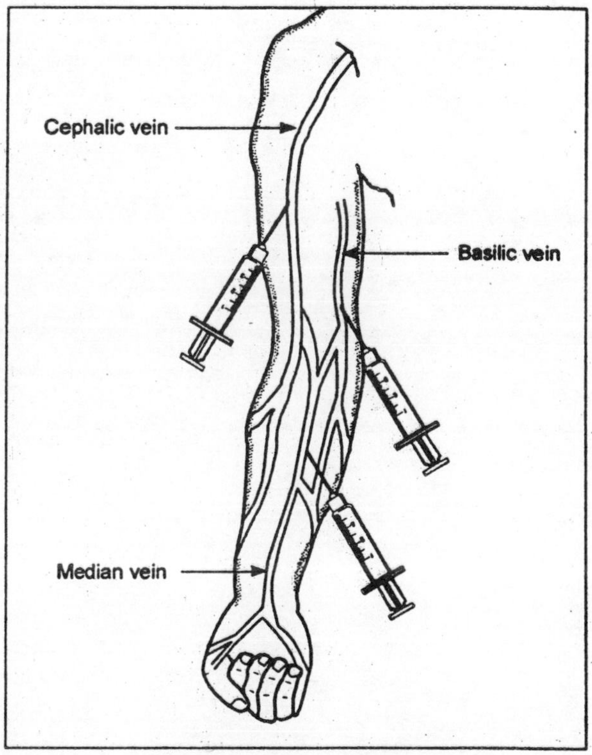

Withdrawal of blood sample

Experiment 44

OBJECT

Withdrawal of blood for clinical haematology and clinical chemistry.

Requirements

Hypodermic needle (18–21 gauge), 70% alcohol, absorbent cotton, tourniquet, container and anticoagulant if needed.

Procedure

Keep the individual in relax position and tie the tourniquet midway between the elbow and shoulder. Select the site and clean it with 70% alcohol. Now the individual is asked to make a fist. Insert the needle into the vein. Blood will flow into the syringe. Collect the required quantity of blood. Now release the tourniquet and withdraw the needle. Transfer the blood into desired container. Record the name of individual, date and time of collection on the lebel of container.

In case of children jugular vein or femoral vein is preferred. The other collecting system is vacutainer which consists of a needle, a needle holder and glass or plastic vacuum tube instead of the syringe barrel and plunger. In this system blood flows automatically into the vacutainer tube so that the need to pull the plunger is avoided. This system is easy to use, quicker and safe.

Result

Name of individual/patient: ______________________ Date: ____________

Age: ______________________________________ Sex: ____________

Amount of blood withdrawn: ____________________ Anticoagulant used: ____________

Vein used: __________________________

Anticoagulant

1. *Salt of EDTA* (1 mg/blood): It is used for blood count, ESR, etc.
2. *Oxalate salts:* Potassium oxalate and ammonium oxalate salts are used together in 2 : 3 ratio respectively, e.g. ESR and haematocrit.
3. *Trisodium citrate* (3.8%): For ESR in 1:4 ratio (citrate : blood).
4. *Heparin* (powder or liquid): For all haematological investigations.
5. *Sodium fluoride* (10 mg/ml of blood): e.g. glucose, urea, creatinine and cholesterol.

Experiment 45

OBJECT

Requirements

Procedure

Result

Experiment 46

OBJECT

Requirements

Procedure

Result

Experiment 47

OBJECT

Requirements

Procedure

Result

VIVA VOCE

Carbohydrates

1. Define and classify carbohydrates.
2. Write the composition of Fehling's solutions (A and B).
3. Write the composition of Benedict's reagent.
4. Why are two Fehling's solutions kept separate?
5. Write the composition of Barfoed's reagent.
6. Which test is given by all carbohydrates?
7. Which test differentiates between fructose and glucose?
8. What are reducing sugars?
9. Which chemical test differentiates lactose from maltose?
10. Which chemical test differentiates starch, dextrin and glycogen?

Proteins and amino acids

1. What are essential amino acids?
2. Classify proteins.
3. Name some chemicals/reagents which identify proteins by precipitation properties.
4. What is biuret test?
5. Benzene ring of the proteins is confirmed by which test?
6. Million's test is applicable to which proteins?
7. Write specific test for peptone.
8. Which colour test is carried out for arginine containing proteins?
9. What is Rosenhim's test?
10. Write biochemical role of proteins in body.

Lipids

1. Classify lipids.
2. Enlist the name of compound lipids.
3. Write biochemical role of lipids in the body.
4. What is emulsification test?
5. What is saponification test?
6. What is grease spot test?
7. What is Salkowski's test?
8. Write specific test for glycerol.
9. Write specific test for cholesterol.

Urine analysis

1. Enlist the normal inorganic constituents of human urine.
2. What are normal organic constituents of human urine?
3. What is haematuria?
4. What are abnormal constituents of human urine?
5. Write clinical significance of the presence of protein in urine.
6. What is glycosuria?
7. What are the causes of glycosuria?
8. Differentiate between diabetes mellitus and diabetes incipidus.
9. What is Rothera's and Benedict's test?
10. What is ketonuria? Write its clinical importance.

. Write clinical importance of bile salts and bile pigments present in human urine.
. Write the clinical importance of urine analysis.
. Name the equipment used in measuring the specific gravity of urine.

nzymology

1. Define and classify enzymes.
2. Write biological importance of enzymes.
3. Write the principle for estimation of diastase content in urine/serum.
4. Write biochemical role of phosphatases.
5. Write clinical importance of acid and alkaline phosphatases.
6. Define apoenzyme and coenzyme.
7. What is king Armstrong unit?
8. What is lipase? How is it estimated?
9. What is SGOT and SGPT?
10. Write the clinical importance of SGOT and SGPT?
11. Write principle for estimation for SGOT and SGPT.
12. Which reaction is catalyzed by SGOT?
13. Why unhemolysed serum should be taken for estimation of SGOT/SGPT?

Clinical chemistry

1. Define biochemistry and pathology.
2. Write the principle of colourimetric method of analysis in clinical biochemistry.
3. What is Beer's law?
4. What is Lambert's law?
5. What is the basic requirement for selection of filter of particular wavelength in colourimetric analysis?
6. Write the basic principle in estimation of blood sugar by *o*-toluidine method.
7. Write the normal range in serum/plasma of the followings—glucose, urea, creatinine, cholesterol, bilirubin.
8. Write clinical importance of urea and creatinine.
9. What are different lipid profiles?
10. Write the principle of cholesterol estimation in serum/plasma.
11. Write the principle of bilirubin estimation in serum/plasma.
12. What is direct and indirect bilirubin?
13. Write the formula for estimation of total bilirubin of serum/plasma.
14. Write formula for estimating serum calcium.
15. Write clinical significance of serum calcium estimation.

Examination of stool and sputum

1. How sputum is collected?
2. Write importance of AFB test of sputum.
3. What parasites are present in human stool?
4. What is Charcot-Leyden and haematoidin crystals? Write their clinical importance.
5. How deposit of parasites by sedimentation technique is prepared?

Withdrawal of blood sample

1. Enlist the different parenteral routes.
2. Write precautions in withdrawal of blood sample by vein puncture.
3. Write the name of common veins for collection of blood sample.
4. What veins are preferred for children for withdrawal of blood sample?
5. Write the name of anticoagulants used in clinical chemistry.

APPENDIX

Manufactures and suppliers of medical diagnostic equipments/reagents/kits, etc.

1. J. Mitra and Co. Ltd.
   A-180, Okhla Industrial Area, Phase 1,
   New Delhi – 110020
2. Mass Diagnostic
   5, Community center, Naraina Industrial Area, Phase 1,
   New Delhi – 110028
3. Miles India Ltd.,
   589, Sayaji pura, Ajwa road,
   Baroda – 390006 (Gujrat)
4. Ranbaxy Diagnostic
   6, Nehru Palace,
   New Delhi – 110019
5. ACE Diagnostic and Biotech Ltd.
   Plot No. 66, Sector 18, Opp. Hipa complex, Huda,
   Gurgaon (Haryana) – 122001
   (Ph: 91-124-5013151, Fax: 91-124-5103829)
6. Span Diagnostic Ltd.
   Plot No. 336, 338, 340, Road no. 3, GIDC,
   Sachin – 394230 (Surat)